SpringerBriefs in Materials

More information about this series at http://www.springer.com/series/10111

Hamid Reza Rezaie · Leila Bakhtiari
Andreas Öchsner

Biomaterials and
Their Applications

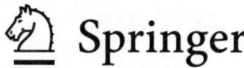 Springer

Hamid Reza Rezaie
Ceramic and Biomaterial Division
Department of Engineering Materials
Iran University of Science and Technology
Tehran
Iran

Leila Bakhtiari
Ceramic and Biomaterial Division
Department of Engineering Materials
Iran University of Science and Technology
Tehran
Iran

Andreas Öchsner
School of Engineering
Griffith University
Southport, QLD
Australia

ISSN 2192-1091   ISSN 2192-1105   (electronic)
SpringerBriefs in Materials
ISBN 978-3-319-17845-5   ISBN 978-3-319-17846-2   (eBook)
DOI 10.1007/978-3-319-17846-2

Library of Congress Control Number: 2015937750

Springer Cham Heidelberg New York Dordrecht London

Printed on acid-free paper

Springer International Publishing AG Switzerland is part of Springer Science+Business Media
(www.springer.com)

Contents

Abstract

Biomaterials are synthetic or natural materials that are used to directly replace, change or improve the living tissues which have been damaged by diseases, trauma, accidents, etc. This biomaterial can be single or in combination with other materials which are used in living tissues at different times. Although a lot of efforts have been done on improving the quality and efficiency of biomaterials, there is a long way to achieve an ideal biomaterial with minimum side effects. This book is an overview of the types of biomaterial (such as bioceramics, biopolymers, metals and biocomposites) and especially nano-biomaterials, their applications in different tissues (drug delivery systems, tissue engineering, implants, etc.) and also to give an overall view in new trends in the biomaterial field the during last decades.

Keywords Biomaterial · Biocompatibility · Tissue engineering · Drug delivery systems · Meso-porous materials · Biocomposite · Surface modification · Implants · Dental material

Chapter 1
Introduction

Biomaterials are synthetic or natural materials intended to function appropriately in a biological environment in which they are used to direct, supplement or replace the functions of living tissues of the human body. After the invention of first generation of materials during 1960–1970 for use inside a human body, synthetic biomaterials became a subject of interest [1]. The use of biomaterials dates back to ancient civilizations. Artificial eyes, ears, teeth and noses were found on Egyptian mummies. Chinese and Indians used waxes, glues, and tissues in reconstructing missing or defective parts of the body. Over the centuries, advancements in synthetic materials, surgical techniques, and sterilization methods have permitted the use of biomaterials in many new ways. Medical practice today utilizes a large number of devices and implants. Biomaterials in the form of implants (sutures, bone plates, joint replacements, ligaments, vascular grafts, heart valves, intraocular lenses, dental implants and etc.) and medical devices (pacemakers, biosensors, artificial hearts, blood tubes and etc.) are widely used to replace and/or restore the function of traumatized or degenerated tissues or organs, to assist in healing, to improve function, to correct abnormalities and then improve the quality of life of the patients.

In the early days all kind of natural materials such as wood, glue and rubber and tissues from living forms and manufactured materials such as iron, zinc, gold and glass were used as biomaterials based on trial and error. The host responses to these materials were extremely varied. Over the last 30 years considerable progress has been made in understanding the interactions between non-living and living materials. Researchers have coined the words "biomaterial" and "biocompatibility" to indicate the biological performance of materials. Materials that are compatible are called biomaterials, and the biocompatibility is a descriptive term which indicates the ability of a material to perform with an appropriate host response, in a specific application. Table 1.1 summarizes various important factors that are considered in selecting material for a biomedical application [2].

© The Author(s) 2015
H. Reza Rezaie et al., *Biomaterials and Their Applications*,
SpringerBriefs in Materials, DOI 10.1007/978-3-319-17846-2_1

Table 1.1 Various factors of importance in material selection for biomedical selection [2]

Factors	Description		
1st level material properties	Chemical/biological characteristics Chemical composition (Bulk and Surface)	Physical characteristic density	Mechanical/structural characteristics Elastic modulus Poisson's ratio Yield strength Tensile strength Compressive strength
2nd level material properties	Adhesion	Surface topology (texture and roughness)	Hardness Shear modulus Shear strength Flexural modulus Flexural strength
Specific functional requirements (based on application)	Biofunctionality (non-thrombogenic, cell adhesion and etc.) Bioinert (non-toxic, non-irritant, non-allergic, non-carcinogenic and etc.) Bioactive Biostability (resistant to corrosion, hydrolysis, oxidation and etc.) Biogradation	Form (solid, porous, coating, film, fiber, mesh, powder) Geometry Coefficient of thermal expansion Electrical conductivity Color, aesthetics Refractive index Opacity or translucency	Stiffness or rigidity Fracture toughness Fatigue strength Creep resistance Friction and wear resistance Adhesion strength Impact strength Proof stress Abrasion resistance
Processing and fabrication	Reproducibility, quality, sterilizability, packaging, secondary processability		
Characteristics of host:	Tissue, organ, species, age, sex, race, health condition, activity, systemic response		
Other	Medical/surgical procedure period of application/ usage cost		

1.1 The History of Biomaterials

The introduction of non-biological materials into the human body took place throughout history. After World War II, the physician was implicitly entrusted with the life and health of the patient and had much more freedom than is seen today to

take heroic action when other options were exhausted. These medical practition-
ers had read about the post-World War II marvels of materials science. Looking at
a patient open on the operating table, they could imagine replacements, bridges,
conduits, and even organ systems based on such materials. Many materials were
tried on the spur of the moment. Some fortuitously succeeded. These were high
risk trials, but usually they took place where other options were not available.

Intraocular lenses, hip and knee prostheses, dental implants, artificial kidney,
artificial hearts, breast implants, vascular grafts, stents, pacemakers, heart valves,
drug delivery systems etc. [3].

1.2   Classification of Biomaterials

The different classes of materials used for the fabrication of bio-implants and
bio-devices can be broadly classified as (1) metallic materials, (2) polymers, (3)
ceramics, (4) composites and (5) natural materials.

1.2.1   Metallic Materials

Metallic materials are most commonly used for load bearing implants and inter-
nal fixation devices. The processing method and purity of the metal determines
its properties. Some featured properties of metallic materials are its high tensile
strength, high yield strength, resistance to cyclic loading (fatigue), resistance to
time dependent deformation (creep) and its corrosion resistance. They generally
find applications in the fabrication of implant devices such as hip joint prosthesis,
knee joint prosthesis, dental implants, cardiovascular devices, surgical instruments
and etc. The most commonly used metals and alloys for medical device applications include stainless steels, commercially pure titanium and its alloys, and
cobalt-based alloys which are briefly discussed below [1].

316L Stainless Steel. Stainless steels are iron based alloys which was first used
in orthopaedic surgery in 1926. These alloys have a minimum of 10.5 % Cr as an
alloying element, needed to prevent the formation of rust. There are two strength-
ening methods for 316L stainless steels: cold-working and controlling grain size.
Each of these methods helps to increase the difficulty of slip of dislocations [3].
Apart from implant applications commercial grade stainless steels are also widely
used for the manufacture of surgical and dental instruments. Although there are
several types of stainless steels (see Table 1.2) in use for medical applications,
316L (18Cr–14Ni–2.5Mo) single phase austenitic (FCC) stainless steel is the
most popular one for implant applications. The "L" in the designation denotes
its low carbon content and as a result it has high corrosion resistance in in-vivo
conditions.

Table 1.2 Types of stainless steels in use for medical applications [1]

Types of stainless steel	Cr content (%)	Medical applications
Martensitic stainless steel	10.5–18	Bone curettes, chisels and gouges, dental burs, dental chisels, curettes, explorers, root elevators and scalers, forceps, hemostats, reactors, orthodontic pliers and scalpels
Ferritic stainless steel	11–30	Solid handles for instruments, guide pins and fasteners
Austenitic stainless steel	16–26	Canulae, dental impression trays, guide pins, hollowware, hypodermic needles, steam sterilizers, storage cabinets, hip implants and knee implants

Cobalt alloys. Among cobalt alloys, Co–Cr based alloys are the most commonly used alloys in biomedical applications. The presence of Cr imparts corrosion resistance and the addition of small amounts of other elements such as iron, molybdenum, or tungsten can make very good high temperature properties and abrasion resistance. Cobalt-based alloys include Haynes-Stellite 21 and 25 (ASTM F75 and F90), forged Co–Cr–Mo alloy (ASTM F799), and multiphase (MP) alloy MP35N (ASTM F562). The F75 and F799 alloys are virtually identical in composition, each being about 58–70 % Co and 26–30 % Cr, with the key difference in their processing history. The other two alloys, F90 and F562, have slightly less Co and Cr, but more Ni (F562) or more tungsten (F90).

Some important clinical applications of these alloys are in dentistry and maxillofacial surgery as partial denture, dental implants, and maxillofacial implants and in orthopaedics as fracture fixation plates and screws and hip and knee prosthesis. Casting Co–Cr-based alloys for the fabrication of implants is not a preferred technique as solidification during casting may result in large dendritic grains and thereby decrease its yield strength. For improving the mechanical properties of these alloys, powder metallurgical techniques such as hot isostatic pressing (HIP) followed by forging [4] have been used for such applications.

Titanium alloys. Commercially pure (CP) titanium (ASTM F67) and extra-low interstitial (ELI) Ti–6Al–4V alloy (ASTM F136) are the two most common titanium-based implant biomaterials. These alloys are suitable for load bearing implants due to its superior mechanical properties (tensile strength and fatigue strength), chemical stability (corrosion resistance), and biocompatibility under in vivo conditions [4–6]. Recent researches showed the dissolution of aluminium and vanadium ions from passivation layer break down during wear in Ti–6Al–4V into the body fluid would have many side effects. Consequently, other titanium alloys such as Ti–6Al–7Nb and Ti–13Nb–13Zr are under study in terms of their corrosion rate, mechanical properties, and biocompatibility as compared to Ti–6Al–4V. Table 1.3 lists titanium and its applications in the biomedical field [1, 3].

Table 1.3 Mechanical properties and clinical applications of Ti-based metallic materials

Alloy	Elastic modulus (GPa)	0.2 % offset yield strength (MPa)	Ultimate tensile strength (MPa)	Elongation (%)	Clinical applications
Pure Ti	102–110	170–480	240–550	15–24	Pacemaker cases, housings for ventricular-assist devices, implantable infusion drug pumps, dental implants, maxillofacial and craniofacial implants, screws and staples for spinal surgery
Ti–6Al–4V	110	860	930	10–15	Total joint replacement arthroplasty primarily for hips and knees
Ti–6Al–7Nb	105	795	860	10	Femoral hip stems, fracture fixation plates, spinal components, fasteners, nails, rods, screws and wire
Ti–13Nb–13Zr	79–84	836–908	973–1037	10–16	Orthopaedic implants

A selection of metallic biomaterials is related to the final application of the bio-medical device, so it is necessary to have adequate information about these materials. Table 1.4 lists the mechanical properties of metallic biomaterials used as implants.

In the titanium based alloys group, there is a special alloy which is known as *Nitinol (Nickel-Titanium Naval Ordnance Laboratory)*. This class of titanium and

Table 1.4 Typical mechanical properties of implant metals [3]

Materials	ASTM designation	Condition	Young's modulus (GPa)	Yield strength (MPa)	Tensile strength (MPa)	Fatigue endurance limit strength (at 10^7 cycles, R $= -1^a$) (MPa)
Stainless steel	F745	Annealed	190	221	483	221–280
	F55, F56, F138, F139	Annealed	190	331	586	241–276
		30 % cold-worked	190	792	930	310–448
		Cold forged	190	1213	1351	820

(continued)

Table 1.4 (continued)

Materials	ASTM designation	Condition	Young's modulus (GPa)	Yield strength (MPa)	Tensile strength (MPa)	Fatigue endurance limit strength (at 10^7 cycles, $R = -1^a$) (MPa)
Co–Cr alloys	F75	As-cast/ annealed	210	448–517	655–889	207–310
		P/M HIP[b]	253	841	1277	725–950
	F799	Hot forged	210	896–1200	1399–1586	600–896
		44 % cold-worked	210	1606	1896	586
	F562	Hot forged	232	965–1000	1206	500
		Cold-worked, aged	232	1500	1795	689–793 (axial tension $R = 0.05$, 30 Hz
Ti alloys	F67	30 % cold-worked Grade 4	110	485	760	300
	F136	Forged annealed	116	896	965	620
		Forged, heat treated	116	1034	1103	620–689

[a]P/M HIP: Powder metallurgy product, hot-isostatically pressed
[b]R is defined as $\sigma_{min}/\sigma_{max}$

nickle alloys in addition to having titanium alloy properties (good mechanical qualities and biocompatibility), have other unique behaviours such as shape memory, extremely high elasticity, force hysteresis, fatigue resistance, thermal deployment, and kink resistance. Clamps for orthopaedic and traumatological bone fixation, filters to retain emboli in vascular surgery, orthodontic wires and heart stents are some important applications of NiTi alloys [3, 7].

1.2.2 Polymers

Polymers are the other category of materials which are used as biomaterials. Polymers are long chain molecules consisting of a large number of small repeating monomers (composer unit). Polymers can be derived either from natural sources or from synthetic organic sources. These materials have already been used in surgical tools, implantable devices, device coatings, catheters, vascular grafts, injectable

Table 1.5 Polymers used as biomaterials [1]

Polymer	Application
Ultrahigh-molecular-weight polyethylene (UHMWPE)	Knee, hip, shoulder joints
Silicone	Finger joints
Polylactic and polyglycolic acid	Sutures
Silicone, acrylic, nylon	Tracheal tubes
Acetal, polyethylene, polyurethane	Heart pacemaker
Polyester, polytetrafluoroethylene, PVC	Blood vessels
Nylon, PVC, silicones	Gastrointestinal segments
Polydimethyl siloxane, polyurethane, PVC	Facial prostheses
Polymethylmethacrylate	Bone cement

biomaterials and therapeutics. Examples of polymers used as biomaterials are listed in Table 1.5. Conducting polymers (CPs) are an important group of polymers that were produced first in 1970s and showed both electrical and optical properties similar to those of metals and inorganic semiconductors, but which also exhibit the attractive properties associated with conventional polymers, such as ease of synthesis and flexibility in processing. Biosensors, neural probes, tissue engineering, drug delivery and bio-actuators are important applications of CPs [1, 8].

Some advantages of using polymers as biomaterials are the easy fabrication and the tuneable surface properties, which can produce a wide range of composites. On the other hand, disadvantages of these biomaterials included: difficulty in sterilization, easy water absorption, weak mechanical properties, and the release of harmful monomers in the human body.

1.2.3 Ceramics

Ceramics are inorganic, nonmetallic materials that have superior compressive strength and biological inertness that make them useful for medical applications. These materials have interatomic bonds (ionic or covalent) which generally form at elevated temperatures. A class of such materials used for skeletal or hard tissue repair are commonly referred to *bioceramics*. These bioceramics may be bioinert (alumina, zirconia), bioresorbable (tricalcium phosphate), bioactive (hydroxyapatite, bioactive glasses, and glass ceramics), or porous for tissue in growth (hydroxyapatite coating, and bioglass coating on metallic materials). Their success depends on their ability to induce bone regeneration and bone in growth at the tissue-implant interface without the intermediate fibrous tissue layer [1, 7].

Depending on the biomaterial type and tissue, different responses occur. Table 1.6 describes these responses.

Ceramics, glasses, and glass-ceramics are widely used in biomedical applications. Drug delivery systems, tissue engineering, dental restoration, implants and

Table 1.6 Responses types of biomaterial-tissue [3]

If the material is toxic, the surrounding tissue dies
If the material is nontoxic and biologically inactive (nearly inert), a fibrous tissue of variable thickness forms
If the material is nontoxic and biologically active (bioactive), an interfacial bond forms
If the material is nontoxic and dissolves, the surrounding tissue replaces it

implant coatings and bone cements are the most important application of biocer-amics. Among the various bioceramics, bioactive ceramics such as hydroxyapatite and bioglass are the most interesting for biomedical applications.

Alumina. Bauxite[1] and native corundum[2] are the main sources of high purity alumina. The most common refining process is the Bayer process, which yields alumina [12]. The Bayer process involves the dissolution of crushed bauxite in sodium hydroxide (NaOH) solution under pressure at high temperatures (up to 300 °C) to form a supersaturated sodium aluminate solution. The hydrated aluminum oxide is precipitated by seeding or as a metastable bayerite on reduction of the pH by carbon dioxide. Washing and dehydrating the precipitate at 1000 ~ 1200 °C turns it into a low-temperature form of "calcined" alumina. Depending on the source of the raw materials other refining processes have been developed. The crystal structure of α-alumina is hexagonal close packed (a = 0.4758 and c = 1.299 nm) and belongs to space group D_3^6d.

The mechanical properties of polycrystalline alumina depend largely on grain size, grain distribution, and porosity. Most alumina used for implant fabrication is either a polycrystalline solid of high density and purity or an artificially grown colourless single crystal similar to sapphire or ruby.

Alumina in general has a hardness of 20 ~ 30 GPa and a Mohs hardness of 9. The high hardness is accompanied by low friction and wear, which are major advantages in using alumina as a joint-replacement material, in spite of its brittleness.

Inertness, biocompatibility, nonsensitization of tissues, excellent wear and friction properties, higher compressive strength to tensile strength make alumina as a good choice for artificial joint and teeth.

Hip joint replacements include 3 parts, the femoral head sphere, the stem or shaft and the cup. The femoral head sphere was made of alumina ceramics and the stem of CoCrMo alloys. The acetabular cup was made of ultra-high molecular weight polyethylene (UHMWPE). There are some problems with this joint replacement technique, such as implant fixation, aseptic loosening, tissue response to wear particulates, infection, ectopic bone formation and pain.

The use of alumina ceramics in other joints (for example in the knee) has been attempted but has not gained much popularity. This is due to the much larger range

---

[1]Hydrated aluminum oxide.

[2]Aluminum oxide mineral (α-alumina).

of motion (ROM) in the knee than in the hip, as well as the much smaller surface contact area and greater incongruency. Again, fixation is much more difficult in the hip than in the knee joint.

In alumina dental implants, fixation is the most difficult problem too. Increasing the surface area, rendering their surface porous, has been tested to solve this problem [9].

Zirconia. Zirconium oxides (zirconia) have been used for the purpose of fabricating implants. Some of their mechanical properties are as good as or better than those of alumina ceramics. They are highly biocompatible, like other ceramics, and can be made into large implants, such as the femoral head of a hip joint replacement. Some of their drawbacks include the fact that they exhibit high density, low hardness, and phase transformations under stress in aqueous conditions, thus degrading their mechanical properties. It is noteworthy that zirconium-niobium metal can be used as an articulating material for joint implants. In bulk behavior this material is very similar to metallic zirconium.

Zircon ($ZrSiO_4$) is the most commercially important zirconium mineral and is found mostly in the mineral baddeleyite. Zircon is a gold-coloured silicate of zirconium, a mineral found in igneous and sedimentary rock and occurring in multi-coloured tetragonal crystals. The transparent varieties are usually deposited in beach sand, and are used as gems. Zircon is first chlorinated to form $ZrCl_4$ in a fluidized bed reactor in the presence of petroleum coke. A second chlorination is required for high-quality zirconium. Zirconium is precipitated with either hydroxides or sulfates, and then is calcined to its oxide [9].

Calcium phosphates. Calcium phosphate (CaP) salts are the major mineral constituents of vertebrate bone and tooth. Within the past 20–30 years interest has intensified in the use of calcium phosphates as biomaterials, but only certain compounds are useful for implantation in the body, since both their solubility and speed of hydrolysis increase with a decreasing calcium/phosphorus ratio. Driessens (1983) stated that those compounds with a Ca/P ratio of less than 1:1 are not suitable for biological implantation [3]. Calcium phosphates show different behavior against microbial attacks, changes in pH and solvent type. Depending on the solvent type, temperature, pressure and impurities, different types of calcium phosphates may be appear. Most common calcium phosphates are listed in Table 1.7.

The biomineral phase, which is one or more types of calcium phosphates, comprises 65–70 % of bone, water accounts for 5–8 % and the organic phase, which is primarily in the form of collagen, accounts for the remaining portion. The collagen, which gives the bone its elastic resistance, acts as a matrix for the deposition and growth of minerals. Among the CaP salts, hydroxyapatite ($Ca_{10}(PO_4)_6(OH)_2$, HAp), as a thermodynamically most stable crystalline phase of CaP in body fluid, possesses the most similarity to the mineral part of bone. It has been well documented that HA can promote new bone ingrowth through osteoconduction mechanism without causing any local or systemic toxicity, inflammation or foreign body response. Currently, HA is commonly the material of choice for various biomedical applications, for example as a replacement for bony and periodontal defects,

Table 1.7 Main calcium phosphates salts [10]

Name	Symbol(s)	Formula	Ca/P
Monocalcium phosphate monohydrate	(MCPM) and (MCPH)	$Ca(H_2PO_4)_2 \cdot H_2O$	0.5
Monocalcium phosphate anhydrous	(MCPA) and (MCP)	$Ca(H_2PO_4)_2$	0.5
Dicalcium phosphate dihydrate (Brushite)	(DCPD)	$CaHPO_4 \cdot 2H_2O$	1.0
Dicalcium phosphate anhydrous (Monetite)	(DCPA) and (DCP)	$CaHPO_4$	1.0
Octacalcium phosphate	(OCP)	$Ca_8(HPO_4)_2(PO_4)_4 \cdot 5H_2O$	1.33
α-Tricalcium phosphate	(α-TCP)	$Ca_3(PO_4)_2$	1.5
β-Tricalcium phosphate	(β-TCP)	$Ca_3(PO_4)_2$	1.5
Amorphous calcium phosphate	(ACP)	$Ca_x(PO4)_y \cdot nH_2O$	1.2–2.2
Hydroxyapatite	(HA) and (HAp)	$Ca_{10}(PO_4)_6(OH)_2$	1.67

Table 1.8 Mechanical properties of hydroxyapatite [3]

Theoretical density	3.156 g cm^3
Hardness	500–800 HV, 2000–3500 Knoop
Tensile strength	40–100 MPa
Bend strength	20–80 MPa
Compressive strength	100–900 MPa
Fracture toughness	$\sim 1 \text{ MPa m}^{0.5}$
Young's modulus	70–120 GPa

alveolar ridge, middle ear implants, tissue engineering systems, drug delivery agent, dental materials and bioactive coating on metallic osseous implants [3, 10]. The main mechanical properties of HA are shown in Table 1.8.

Hydroxyapatite can be synthesized by different methods. Dry methods, wet methods and high temperature methods are the most important category of HA synthesizing methods. Table 1.9 summarizes these methods in details. By using different methods, different types of HA with different properties were formed.

In dry methods there is not a solvent during the synthesis and the two main methods of this category are solid-state synthesis and the mechanochemical process. These methods have the convenience of producing highly crystalline HA from relatively inexpensive raw materials. The main disadvantage is the large size of particles in the case of solid-state synthesis and the low phase purity of HA in the case of the mechanochemical process.

In wet methods, various sources of calcium and phosphates ions were used. Conventional chemical precipitation, hydrolysis method, sol–gel method, hydrothermal method, emulsion method, and sonochemical method are common routes of wet methods. In wet methods there is exact control on the morphology and size especially in synthesize of nanosized particles but there are some difficulties in crystallinity and phase purity control.

Table 1.9 Comparison of different methods of HA synthesis [10]

Method		Morphology	Crystallinity degree	Phase purity	Ca/P ratio	Size	Size distribution
Dry methods	Solid-state method	Diverse	Very high	Usually low	Variable	Usually micron	Wide
	Mechanochemical method	Diverse	Very high	Low	Usually non-stoichiometric	Nano	Usually wide
Wet methods	Chemical precipitation	Diverse	Frequently low	Variable	Non-stoichiometric	Usually nano	Variable
	Hydrolysis method	Diverse	Variable	Usually high	Stoichiometric	Variable	Variable
	Sol–gel method	Diverse	Variable (usually low)	Variable	Stoichiometric	Nano	Narrow
High temperature methods	Hydrothermal method	Frequently needle-like	Very high	Usually high	Stoichiometric	Nano or micron	Usually wide
	Emulsion	Frequently needle-like	Frequently low	Variable	Non-stoichiometric	Nano	Narrow
	Sonochemical method	Diverse (usually needle-like)	Variable	Usually high	Variable	Nano	Usually narrow
	Combustion method	Diverse (usually irregular)	Variable	Usually high	Variable	Usually nano	Wide
	Pyrolysis method	Diverse	High	variable	Usually stoichiometric	Nano particles embedded in micron aggregates	Variable
	Synthesis from biogenic sources	Diverse	Variable	Usually high	Variable	Variable	Variable
	Combination procedures	Diverse (frequently needle-like)	Frequently high	Usually high	Usually stoichiometric	Usually nano	Variable

Table 1.10 Commercial biphasic calcium phosphates and their composites [16]

HA/β-TCP ratio	Commercial name
60/40; 20/80	MBCP® (Biomatlante, France)
20/80	Tribone 80® (Strycker Europe)
60/40	Osteosynt® (Einco Ltd, Brazil)
60/40	Triosite® (Zimmer, IND)
60/40	4Bone® (MIS Israel)
60/40	OptiMX® (Exactech USA)
55/45	Eurocer 400® (Depuy-Bioland, France)
65/35	Eurocer 200® (Depuy-Bioland, France)
Composites	
BCP/collagen	Allograft (Zimmer, IN)
BCP/HPMC	MBCP Gel® (Biomatlante France)
BCP/fibrin	Tricos® (Baxter Biosciences Biosurgery)
BCP/silicon	FlexHA (Xomed, FL)
Calcium phosphate cement	MCPCTM (Biomatlante France)

In the high temperature process, high crystallinity and good chemical homogeneity will be achieved but there is poor control on the variables.

Synthesis from biogenic sources included using natural materials such as bone waste, eggshells, exoskeletons of marine organisms, naturally derived biomolecules, and bio-membranes. The main disadvantage of this method is producing large size particles.

Combination procedures include two or more distinct methods in HA synthesis. Hydrothermal-mechanochemical, hydrothermal-hydrolysis, and hydrothermal-micro-emulsion have received more attention among researchers. However other combination methods such as microwave combination with other methods were also investigated [10].

Tricalcium phosphate/hydroxyapatite (BCP[3]). The term biphasic calcium phosphate (BCP) was first used by Ellinger et al. to describe the bio-ceramic previously described as "tricalcium phosphate" but was shown by LeGeros in 1986 using X-ray diffraction (XRD) to consist of a mixture of 80 % HA and 20 % β-TCP. LeGeros, Daculsi et al. reported that the bioactivity of these ceramics may be controlled by manipulating the HA/β-TCP ratios [11–15]. Now commercial BCPs are available for dental and orthopedic applications (see Table 1.10).

BCP ceramics were formed in different shapes for different applications, such as blocks, granules, cone etc. Combination of these particles with polymers can make BCP composites. Main application of BCP ceramics are bone tissue engineering scaffolds, bone regeneration, gene therapy and drug delivery systems.

---

[3]Biphasic Calcium Phosphate.

BCP ceramics can produced by sintering of synthetic calcium deficient appatites (CDAs) above 900 °C according to the following reaction:

$$Ca_{10-X}M_X(PO_4)_{6-y}(HPO_4)_y(OH)_2 \rightarrow Ca_{10}(PO_4)_6(OH)_2 + Ca_3(PO_4)_2$$

CDAs may be represented by the formula $Ca_{10-X}M_X(PO_4)_{6-y}(HPO_4)_y$ where M represents other ions (sodium, magnesium) that can substitute for calcium (Ca) ions. CDAs can be obtained by precipitation, hydrolysis of non-apatite calcium phosphate and mechanically mixing of HA and TCP [16].

- *Degradation rate of calcium phosphates*:

Biodegradation of calcium phosphate ceramics depended on a few factors. As a result, the biodegradation rate increases as:

1. Surface area increases (powders > porous solid > dense solid);
2. Crystallinity decreases;
3. Crystal perfection decreases;
4. Crystal and grain size decrease;
5. There are ionic substitutions of $CO^{-3}{}_2$, Mg^{2+}, and Sr^{2+} in HA.

Factors that have an effect on the decreasing rate of biodegradation include:
(1) F^- substitution in HA; (2) Mg^{2+} substitution in β-TCP; and (3) lower β-TCP/HA ratios in biphasic calcium phosphates.

Bioglass, bioactive glass-ceramic. Bioactive glasses are amorphous silicate-based materials which are compatible with the human body, bond to bone and can stimulate new bone growth while dissolving over time. They therefore have the potential of bone regeneration. Insoluble porous glasses have been used as carriers for enzymes, antibodies, and antigens, offering the advantages of resistance to microbial attacks, pH changes, solvent conditions, temperature, and packing under high pressure required for rapid flow. Insoluble glasses have also been developed as a microinjectable delivery system for radioactive isotopes for in situ treatment of tumors. The glass microspheres go to the site of the tumor by way of the blood supply, and the radiation kills the cancer cells with very little damage to the other tissues, saving thousands of patients [3, 16].

Common characteristics of bioactive glasses and bioactive ceramics is forming a biologically-active carbonated HA layer (HCA) that provides the bonding interface with tissues. There are three key compositional features to these bioactive glasses that distinguish them from traditional soda-lime-silica glasses:
(1) Less than 60 mol% SiO_2; (2) High Na_2O and CaO content; and (3) a high CaO/P_2O_5 ratio. These features make the surface highly reactive when it is exposed to an aqueous medium [3].

The original bio-glass was produced by melt-processing, which involves melting high-purity oxides (SiO_2, Na_2CO_3, $CaCO_3$ and P_2O_5) in a crucible in a furnace at 1370 °C. Platinum crucibles must be used to ensure there is no contamination of the glass. The bio-glass particulate is made by pouring the melt into water to quench, creating a frit. The frit is then dried and ground to the desired particle size range. Bio-glass can also be poured into pre-heated (350 °C) moulds (graphite) to produce rods or as-cast components. Although calcium and phosphate components were in the glass composition because of their presence in bone, soda was added merely to reduce the melting point of the system so that it could be melted in a conventional furnace [16].

Bioactive glass-ceramics are similar to bioactive glass with less than phosphor pentoxide (P_2O_5) and more than sodium oxide (Na_2O). Hench et al. (1972) showed that some $Na_2O–CaO–SiO_2–P_2O_5$ glasses bond to living bone without forming fibrous tissue around them which was known as Bio-glass®, but their low mechanical strength forced researchers to use various types of glass precipitating different crystalline phases to improve their mechanical strength, known as glass-ceramics [16].

Many bioactive silica glasses are based upon a formula called 45S5, signifying 45 wt% SiO_2 and 5:1 ratio of CaO to P_2O_5. Table 1.11 listed the major bioactive glass and glass ceramics. Ceravital®, which precipitates apatite in $Na_2O–K_2O–MgO–CaO–SiO_2–P_2O_5$ glass, glass-ceramic A-W, which precipitates apatite and wollastonite in $MgO–CaO–SiO_2–P_2O_5$glass, Bioverit®, which precipitates apatite and phlogopite in $Na_2O–MgO–CaO–Al_2O_3–SiO_2–P_2O_5–F$ glass, Ilmaplant®, which precipitates apatite and wollastonite in $Na_2O–K_2O–MgO–CaO–SiO_2–P_2O_5–CaF_2$ glass (Berger et al. 1989) and glass-ceramics that precipitate canasite in $Na_2O–K_2O–CaO–CaF_2P_2O_5–SiO_2$ glass are examples. Among these, glass-ceramic A-W has been the most widely used clinically [16].

The fabrication process of bioactive glass-ceramics is similar to that of bio-glasses which certain types of glass can give a composite in which one or more types of crystalline particles are homogeneously dispersed in a glassy matrix when it is subjected to an appropriate heat treatment. Most bioactive glass and glass ceramics are listed in Table 1.11 [16].

1.2.4 Composites

The word composite means "consisting of two or more distinct parts". Composites consist of two phases, one continuous phase which is called the matrix and one discontinuous phase which is called the reinforcement. Different reinforcements and matrixes make different composites. Mainly factors that affected composite structure are:

- Shape, size and distribution of reinforcement;
- Reinforcement properties and volume percentage;
- Bioactivity of the reinforcement;
- Matrix properties such as molecular weight and grain size;
- Reinforcement-matrix interfacial state.

Some promising medical applications of biomedical composites include their use in total joint replacements, spine rods, discs, plates, dental posts, screws, ligaments and catheters.

Table 1.11 Major bioactive glass and glass ceramics (weight percent) [3]

	45S5 bioglass	45S5F bioglass	45S5.4F bioglass	40S5B5 bioglass	52S4.6 bioglass	55S4.3 bioglass	KGC ceravital	KGS ceravital	KGy213 ceravitl	A-W GC	MB GC
SiO_2	45	45	45	40	52	55	46.2	46	38	34.2	19–52
P_2O_5	6	6	6	6	6	6				16.3	4–24
CaO	24.5	12.25	14.7	24.5	21	19.5	20.2	33	31	44.9	9–3
$Ca(PO_3)_2$							25.5		13.5		
CaF_2		12.25	9.8							0.5	
MgO							2.9			4.6	5–15
MgF_2											
Na_2O	24.5	24.5	24.5	24.5	21	19.5	4.8	5	4		3–5
K_2O							0.4				3–5
Al_2O_3								7			12–33
B_2O_3				5							
Ta_2O_5/TiO_2								6.5			
Structure	G[a]	G	G	G			G-C[b]	G-C		G-C	G-C

[a] G Glass
[b] G-C Glass-Ceramic

The main reinforcing materials that have been used in biomedical composites are carbon fibers, polymer fibers, ceramic particles and glass fibers with particles. Depending upon the application, the reinforcements have either been inert or absorbable. Several nanocomposites have also been studied in the last few years that contain carbon nanotubes, nanoclays, silica, and hydroxyapatite nanoparticles [1, 3].

1.2.5 Natural Materials

Natural materials are mainly natural polymers such as collagen and glycosaminoglycans which are used in clinical applications. Collagen is a fibrous protein that connects and supports other bodily tissues such as skin, bone, tendons, muscles, and cartilage. It is the most plentiful available protein present in the bodies of mammals, including humans. Glycosaminoglycan is the most abundant heteropolysaccharide present in the body. Glycosaminoglycans occur primarily on the surface of cells or in the extracellular matrix (ECM). These materials showed some advantages: similarity to macromolecular substances and easy recognition by the biological environment, non-toxicity and biodegradability are important advantages of these materials [1].

1.3 Biocompatibility

A biomaterial is defined as a material that can be used in human tissues without causing any harmful effects. Biocompatibility is a word which is used to speak about biomaterials and defined as the ability of a material to exist in the human body and the compatibility of these.

Biocompatibility has traditionally been concerned with implantable devices that have been intended to remain within an individual for a long time. During the years 1940 and 1980, the first generation of implantable devices were investigated and as a result they discovered that materials that were the least chemically reactive were the most biocompatible.

Three factors should be considered in the use of biomaterials and its biocompatibility investigation. The first was that the response to specific individual materials could vary from one application site to another. Thus biocompatibility could not solely be dependent on the material characteristics but also had to be defined by the situation in which the material is used. Secondly, an increasing number of applications required that the material should specifically react with the tissues rather than be ignored by them, as required in the case of an inert material. Thirdly, some applications required that the material should degrade over time in the body rather than remain indefinitely.

Accordingly, biocompatibility was redefined in 1987 as follows:

Biocompatibility refers to the ability of a material to perform with an appropriate host response in a specific situation.

Table 1.12   Major material variables that could influence the host response [17]

Bulk material composition, micro- (or nano)-structure, morphology
Crystallinity and crystallography
Elastic constants
Water content, hydrophobic–hydrophilic balance
Macro-, micro-, nano-porosity
Surface chemical composition, chemical gradients, surface molecular mobility
Surface topography
Surface energy
Surface electrical/electronic properties
Corrosion parameters, ion release profile, metal ion toxicity (for metallic materials)
Degradation profile, degradation product form and toxicity (for polymeric materials)
Leachables, additives, catalysts, contaminants and their toxicity (for polymeric materials)
Dissolution/degradation profile, degradation product toxicity (for ceramic materials)
Wear debris release profile

There are some material variables that could influence the host response. The most important variables are described in Table 1.12.

Parameters that can be significant in biocompatibility expression:

- *Implant location*: Being at surface or at depth of a tissue is effective in biocompatibility. Subcutaneously, intradermal, intramuscular or intraosseous implants show different effects in human body.
- *Design based on the application*: Try to use materials that comply with the requirements of the target tissue.
- *Shape of the biomaterial*: Biomaterial shape affects its biocompatibility in the body and environment (smooth surfaces, shapes with irregular angles…)
- *Move according to the application*: In the case that the biomaterial must perform movement, the durability, fatigue, abrasion and other mechanical properties must be considered. For example, in heart valve design, erosion of the valve is the most common cause of damage. So it is necessary to consider the type of the biomaterial within the application.
- *Time duration of application*
- *Biological condition of the patient*
- *Physical and chemical properties of biomaterial*

References

1. Paital SR, Dahotre NB (2009) Calcium phosphate coatings for bio-implant applications: materials, performance factors, and methodologies. Mater Sci Eng R Rep 66(1):1–70
2. Ramakrishna S, Mayer J, Wintermantel E, Leong KW (2001) Biomedical applications of polymer-composite materials: a review. Compos Sci Technol 61(9):1189–1224
3. Ratner BD, Hoffman AS, Schoen FJ (2013) Biomaterials science an introduction to materials in medicine, 3rd edn. Elsevier Ltd, Amsterdam

4. Niinomi M (2002) Recent metallic materials for biomedical applications. Metall Mater Trans A 33(3):477–486
5. Aparicio C, Gil FJ, Fonseca C, Barbosa M, Planell JA (2003) Corrosion behaviour of commercially pure titanium shot blasted with different materials and sizes of shot particles for dental implant applications. Biomaterials 24(2):263–273
6. Van Noort R (1987) Titanium: the implant material of today. J Mater Sci 22(11):3801–3811
7. Binyamin G, Shafi BM, Mery CM (2006) Biomaterials: a primer for surgeons. Semin Pediatr Surg 15(4):276–283
8. Guimard NK, Gomez N, Schmidt CE (2007) Conducting polymers in biomedical engineering. Prog Polym Sci 32(8):876–921
9. Park JB (2008) Bioceramics: properties, characterizations, and applications, vol 218, Springer, New York
10. Sadat-Shojai M, Khorasani M-T, Dinpanah-Khoshdargi E, Jamshidi A (2013) Synthesis methods for nanosized hydroxyapatite of diverse structures. Acta Biomater 9(8):7591–7621
11. Nery EB, Lee KK, Czajkowski S, Dooner JJ, Duggan M, Ellinger RF, Henkin JM, Hines R, Miller M, Olson JW (1990) A veterans administration cooperative study of biphasic calcium phosphate ceramic in periodontal osseous defects. J Periodontol 61(12):737–744
12. LeGeros RZ, Lin S, Rohanizadeh R, Mijares D, LeGeros JP (2003) Biphasic calcium phosphate bioceramics: preparation, properties and applications. J Mater Sci Mater Med 14(3):201–209
13. Daculsi G, Passuti N (1990) Effect of the macroporosity for osseous substitution of calcium phosphate ceramics. Biomaterials 11:86
14. Yamamuro T, Hench LL, Wilson J (1990) CRC handbook of bioactive ceramics. CRC press, Boca Raton
15. Daculsi G, Passuti N, Martin S, Deudon C, LeGeros RZ, Raher S (1990) Macroporous calcium phosphate ceramic for long bone surgery in humans and dogs. Clinical and histological study. J Biomed Mater Res 24(3):379–396
16. Kokubo T, Kaisha NMMK (2008) Bioceramics and their clinical applications. Woodhead Publication and Maney Publication, Cambridge and Leeds
17. Williams DF (2008) On the mechanisms of biocompatibility. Biomaterials 29(20):2941–2953

Chapter 2
Application of Biomaterials

The main applications of biomaterials can be classified into the categories below and described later:

- Cardiovascular medical devices (stents, grafts and etc.)
- Orthopedic and dental applications (implants, tissue engineered scaffolds and etc.)
- Ophthalmologic applications (contact lenses, retinal prostheses and etc.)
- Bioelectrodes and biosensors
- Burn dressings and skin substitutes
- Sutures
- Drug delivery systems

Cardiovascular medical devices. Heart valves, endovascular stents, vascular grafts, stent grafts and other cardiovascular grafts are common medical devices in cardiovascular applications. There are several major forms of valvular heart disease, most involving the aortic and/or the mitral valve. The most common type of valve disease and most frequent indication for valve replacement overall is calcific aortic stenosis obstruction at the aortic valve secondary to age-related calcification of the cusps of a valve that was previously anatomically normal. In case of vascular pathologies, stents and vascular graft is used. Different polymers and metals with or without coating can be applied in this category (titanium, polytetrafluoroethylene and etc.) [1].

Tissue engineering scaffolds. Tissue engineering is one of the most important ways to achieve tissues for repair or replacement applications. Its goal is to design and fabricate reproducible, bioactive and bioresorbable 3D scaffolds with tailored properties that are able to maintain their structure and integrity for predictable times, even under load-bearing conditions. Scaffolds can be applied in different tissues. It is only important to note that it only in designing the scaffold, type of fabrication and biomaterial selection depending on the target organ and its cells that can be affected on final application. Chemistry, architecture, porosity and rate of degradation should provide a sufficient mechanical environment and should facilitate cell attachment, proliferation and migration, waste nutrient exchange, vascularization and tissue ingrowth. Also there should be a proper ratio between degradation of the scaffold and tissue ingrowth [2].

© The Author(s) 2015
H. Reza Rezaie et al., *Biomaterials and Their Applications*,
SpringerBriefs in Materials, DOI 10.1007/978-3-319-17846-2_2

There are various types of scaffold fabrication methods. At first, only polymeric scaffolds were used but gradually composite scaffolds and especially ceramic/polymer scaffolds have been used. The main important scaffold fabrication methods are: fiber bonding, solvent casting and particulate leaching, compression molding, extrusion, freeze-drying, phase emulsion, solid free form fabrication and electrospinning. Differences between these methods are temperature, pressure, solvent type, porogen (which is responsible for making pores) and etc.

Recently researchers used mesostructured materials in scaffolds to supply drug and biological agents in situ during degradation of scaffold and growing new tissue.

Ophthalmologic applications. Vision impairment/low vision, blindness, refractive error (Myopia and Hyperopia), astigmatism, presbyopia, cataracts, primary open-angle glaucoma, age-related macular degeneration (AMD) and diabetic retinopathy are common ophthalmologic diseases. To improve the life of these patients, many implants have been applied. The main biomaterials which are used in this category are summarized in Table 2.1 [1].

Bioelectrodes and biosensors. Bioelectrodes are sensors used to transmit information into or out of the body. Surface or transcutaneous electrodes used to monitor or measure electrical events that occur in the body are considered monitoring or recording electrodes. Typical applications for recording electrodes include electrocardiography, electroencephalography, and electromyography information into or out of the body. Various parameters influence the material selection of electrodes (see Table 2.2).

These bioelectrodes are mainly applied in cardiology and neurology applications. A biosensor is a sensor that uses biological molecules, tissues, organisms or principles to measure chemical or biochemical concentrations. Biosensors can

Table 2.1 Ophthalmic implant materials commonly used [1]

Implant	Materials which used
Contact lenses	Poly(methyl methacrylate) (PMMA), 2-hydroxyethyl methacrylate (HEMA) copolymers, silicone hydrogels
Inlays or onlays	Hydrogels, collagen, permeable membranes
Intraocular lenses	Optic: PMMA, hydrophobic acrylic, silicone, hydrophilic acrylic Haptic: polypropylene, PMMA, polyimide, polyvinylidene fluoride (PVDF)
Ophthalmic viscosurgical device (OVD)	Chrondroitin sulfate, sodium hyaluronate, hyaluronic acid, hydroxypropyl methylcellulose (HPMS), polyacrylamide, collagen, or combinations of these materials
Glaucoma shunts	Plates: silicone (impregnated with barium), polypropylene Tubing: silicone
Vitreous replacements	Silicone oil, gases

Table 2.2 Parameters influencing the material selection of electrodes [1]

Electrode	Surface area, geometry, and surface condition
Electrical	Potential, current, and quantity of charge
Environmental	Mass-transfer variables and solution variables
Engineering	Availability, cost, strength, and fabricability

be used in many medical and non-medical applications. Biomedical sensors are sensors that detect medically relevant parameters; these could range from simple physical parameters like blood pressure or temperature, to analyses for which biosensors are appropriate (e.g. blood glucose). Biosensors can work by changes in pH, ions, blood gases (O_2, CO_2 and etc.), drugs, hormones, proteins, viruses, bacteria, tumors and etc. [1].

Burn dressing and skin substitutes. Skin is the largest organ that protects body from microorganisms and external forces, integrates complex sensory nervous and immune systems, controls fluid loss, and serves important aesthetic function. Deep skin injuries due to deep cuts, burns or degloving injuries can cause significant physiological derangement, expose the body to a risk of systemic infection, and become a life threatening problem. So the need of skin substitutes depending on wound depth is felt. An ideal skin substitute must be inexpensive, long lasting, a bacterial barrier, semipermeable to water, elastic, easy to apply, painless to the patient, non-antigenic and non-toxic and has durable shelf-time. Today a lot of commercial skin substitutes are applied [1].

Sutures. Suture is any strand of material that is used to ligate blood vessels or approximate tissue. Ligatures are used to achieve hemostasis or to close a structure to prevent leakage. The suture device is comprised of: the suture strand; the surgical needle; and the packaging material used to protect the suture and needle during storage. The ideal suture must be biocompatible, sterile, compliant, adequate knot/ straight strength, secure and stable knot, strength and mass loss profiles adequate for proposed usage, low friction, adequate needle attachment strength, atraumatic needle design, non-electrolytic, non-capillary, non-allergenic, non-carcinogenic, minimally reactive, uniform and predictable performance. Silk, nylon, polyester, cotton, polypropylene, ultra-high molecular weight polyethylene (UHMWPE), stainless steel and synthetic absorbable polymers such as poly glicolic acid (PGA), p-dioxanone (PDO) and etc. are the main materials that are used as sutures yet [1].

Drug delivery systems (***DDS***). Drug delivery systems introduced as formulations or instruments which enable to control the release rate of a biological agent (especially a drug) in the target site. Drug delivery systems are an interface between patient and drug. Drugs can be introduced to the organ by different anatomical routes due to disease and drug type: Digestive system (oral, anal), oral, rectal, parenteral (subcutaneous, intramuscular, intravenous, arterial), mucous membranes, respiratory tract by inhalation, subcutaneous or intraosseous are man anatomical routes.

By increasing the size the dosage in single dose administration, side effects would appear so in order to reduce these side effects, coatings with varying thickness, are

Table 2.3   DDS systems [1]

Macroscale DDS ("zero order" constant delivery rate DDS)   • Implants (e.g. subcutaneous or intramuscular)   • Inserts (e.g. vaginal, ophthalmic)   • Ingested DDS (e.g. osmotic pumps, hydrogels)   • Topical DDS (e.g. skin patches)
Macroscale and microscale DDS (site-specific, sustained delivery rate DDS)   • Surface-coated DDS (e.g. oral tablets, catheters, drug-eluting stents)   • Injected DD depots (e.g. degradable microparticles and phase separated masses)
Nanoscale DDS (targeted DDS)   • Injected nanocarrier DDS (e.g. PEGylated drugs, polymer-drug conjugates, PEGylated liposomes, PEGylated polymeric micelles, and drug nanoparticles, sometimes targeted by monoclonal antibodies or cell membrane receptor ligands)

applied. Such formulations are now known as "sustained release" or "prolonged release" products. However, the pharmacokinetics of such products depended greatly on the local in vivo patient environment and as such, vary from patient to patient. These systems are called "zero order" systems because they release drug during time in a constant rate. These reasons were among the most important driving forces that led to the birth of the field of "controlled drug delivery" (CDD) in the mid to late 1960s that became known as "macro-scale devices" that exhibit constant or zero order drug delivery rates, leading to constant plasma drug concentrations over long time durations of drug delivery. By the rapid growth of nanoscale materials, injectable targeting drug delivery systems appear (see Table 2.3) [1].

Dental materials. Restorative materials have been used as tooth crowns and root replacements. Four groups of materials which are used in dentistry today are metals, ceramics polymers and composites. Despite recent advances in material science and dentistry, there still is not a proper material for restorative dentistry. Characteristics of an ideal restorative material are listed below:

- Be biocompatible
- Bond permanently to tooth structure or bone
- Match the natural appearance of tooth structure and other visible tissues
- Exhibit properties similar to those of tooth enamel, dentin and other tissues
- Be capable of initiating tissue repair or regeneration of missing or damaged tissue

Dental materials can be classified in two categories: preventive materials, restorative material. Preventive dental materials include pit and fissure sealants, sealing agents that prevent leakage, materials that are used primarily for the antibacterial effects, liners, bases, cements and restorative materials that are used primarily because the release fluoride, chlorhexidine or other therapeutic agents used to prevent or inhibit the progression of tooth decay. This type of materials used for short-term application. Restorative dental materials consist of all synthetic components that can be used to repair or replace tooth structure, including primes, bonding agents, liners, cement bases, amalgams, resin based composites, compomers, metal-ceramics, hybrid ionomers, cast metals and denture polymers. Restorative materials can be used for both short and long-term applications. Restorative materials can be classified as *direct restorative materials* and *indirect restorative materials* dependent on whether they are used. Direct fabricated intraorally and indirect fabricated extraorally [3].

Because of importance of restorative dental materials, explain more about this part. Dental amalgam has been used traditionally for filling dental cavities. Amalgam is a mixture of copper, tin, zinc, mercury, silver and other trace metals. Later cement dental restorative materials were used as restorative materials. To achieve adhesive bonding in the general case of two rigid solids, such as a tooth enamel surface and an orthodontic bracket, it is necessary to apply a fluid adhesive between them.

Moreover, the fluid must be of appropriate chemical formulation to initially wet both surfaces, exhibiting a low contact angle. One or both surfaces may have been subjected to some form of pre-treatment or conditioning with an etchant or primer that, inter alia, may have modified surface porosity. In this case, the adhesive fluid may be drawn into the solid surface layers by capillary action. The presence of a suitable fluid between two solids greatly enhances the potential for intermolecular force interactions at each solid–fluid boundary.

Dental cements can be classified to:

- Conventional acid-base cements
- Poly-electrolyte cements: Zinc poly carboxylates and glass ionomers
- Resin-modified glass-ionomer cements
- Dual-setting resin-based cements

Conventional acid-base cements

Dental cements are, traditionally, fast-setting pastes obtained by mixing solid and liquid components. Most of these materials set by an acid-base reaction, and subsequently developed resin cements harden by polymerization. They have various compositions. This material is composed primarily of zinc oxide powder and a 50 % phosphoric acid solution containing aluminum and zinc. The mixed material sets to a hard, rigid cement by formation of an amorphous zinc phosphate binder. The bonding arises entirely from penetration into mechanically produced irregularities on the surface of the prepared tooth and the fabricated restorative material. Classifications of dental cements are summarized in Table 2.4.

Poly-electrolyte cements: Zinc poly carboxylates and glass ionomers

Poly (carboxylic acid) cements were developed in 1967 to provide materials with properties comparable to those of phosphate cements, but with adhesive properties of calcified tissues. This type of cement is composed of zinc oxide and aqueous poly (acrylic acid) solution. The metal ion cross-links the polymer structure via carboxyl groups, and other carboxyl group's complex to Ca ions in the surface of the tissue. Adequate physical properties, excellent biocompatibility in the tooth, and adhesion to enamel and dentin are main advantages of these cements being opaque is the main problem with these cements. The need for a translucent material led to the development of the glass-ionomer cements (GIC). GICs are also based on poly (acrylic acid) or its copolymers with itaconic or maleic acids, but

Table 2.4 Classification of dental cements [1]

Dental cements	Components	Setting mechanism
Zinc phosphate	Zinc oxide powder, phosphoric acid liquid	Acid–base reactions; Zn complexation
Zinc polycarboxylate	Zinc oxide powder, aqueous poly(acrylic acid)	Acid–base reactions; Zn complexation
Glass ionomer (polyalkenoate)	Ca, Sr, Al silicate glass powder aqueous poly(acrylic acid-itaconic acid)	Acid–base reactions; Metal ion complexation
Resin modified glass ionomer	Dimethacrylate monomers. Aqueous poly(acrylic acid methacrylate) co-monomers. Silicate or other glass fillers	Peroxide-amine or photo-initiated polymerization
Resin-based	Aromatic or urethane dimethacrylates, HEMA	Photoinitiated addition polymerization
Dentin adhesive	Etchant: Phosphoric acid (aq.) Primer: HEMA in ethanol or acetone Bond resin: Dimethacrylate monomers	Photoinitiated addition polymerization

utilize a calcium aluminosilicate glass powder instead of zinc oxide. GICs set by cross-linking of the polyacid with calcium and aluminum ions from the glass, together with formations of a silicate gel structure.

Resin-modified glass-ionomer cements

Polyacid molecules contain both ionic carboxylate and polymerizable methacrylate groups. It is induced to set by both an acid-base reaction and visible light polymerization. Adhesive bonding but not complete sealing is obtained, because of the imperfect adaptation to the bonded surfaces under practical conditions.

Dual-setting resin-based cements

Dual-setting resin-based cements are fluid or paste-like monomer systems based on aromatic or urethane dimethacrylates. They are normally consisting of two-component materials that are mixed to induce setting. They may also be light-cured. These set materials are strong, hard, rigid, insoluble and cross-linked polymers [1].

References

1. Lemons JE, Ratner BD, Hoffman AS, Schoen FJ (2013) Biomaterials science an introduction to materials in medicine, 3rd edn. Elsevier Ltd, Amsterdam
2. Holzapfel BM, Reichert JC, Schantz JT, Gbureck U, Rackwitz L, Nöth U, Jakob F, Rudert M, Groll J, Hutmacher DW (2012) How smart do biomaterials need to be?—a translational science and clinical point of view. Adv Drug Deliv Rev 65(4):581–603
3. Anusavice KJ (2003) Phillips' science of dental materials. Elsevier Health Sciences

Chapter 3
Bio-implants and Bio-devices

A proper design of an implant material is aimed to provide the required durability, functionality and biological response. Durability and functionality depends on the bulk properties of the material, whereas biological response depends on the surface chemistry, surface topography, surface roughness, wettability, surface charge, and surface energy. Biocompatible implant materials should be nontoxic, noncarcinogenic, with little or no foreign body reaction and be chemically stable or corrosion resistant.

The main roles of orthopaedic implant devices is to restore the function of load-bearing joints which are subjected to high level of mechanical stresses, wear, and fatigue in the course of normal activity. Prostheses for hip, knee, ankle, shoulder and elbow joints are important orthopedic implants. They also need devices such as wires, pins, plates, screws and etc. for fracture fixation. Metals (Ti–6Al–4V, Co–Cr–Mo, stainless steel), polymers [poly(methyl methacrylate) (PMMA)], ultrahigh-molecular-weight polyethylene (UHMWPE), and ceramics (alumina, zirconia, hydroxyapatite) are the three classes of materials that are most commonly used for fabricating orthopedic implants. Depending on the biomaterial type that is used for implant fabrication, sometimes coating implants is necessary. Coating materials should be biocompatible, non-toxic, non-mutagen, non-allergic and also stability in chemical and corrosion conditions.

Treatment of heart problems is done by cardiovascular devices. Due to rhythmic expansion and contraction of the heart to supply blood to different organs of the body, significant attention is needed in cardiovascular devices design. After several years of its function, this may result in a structural change in the valve and thereby it may not open and close fully. Cardiovascular devices and pace makers are commonly used devices in treatment of heart problems.

Ophthalmic devices such as intraocular lenses (IOL) used to help patients with cataract or visual disability. Dental implants are devices which are used to replacing both tooth and root. Wound healing involves the use of alternate skin substitutes to treat patients suffering from severe burns, injuries, chronic nonhealing ulcers and etc. The other category of bio-devices are drug delivery systems that are used for controlled and targeted delivery of drugs to the body [1].

© The Author(s) 2015
H. Reza Rezaie et al., *Biomaterials and Their Applications*,
SpringerBriefs in Materials, DOI 10.1007/978-3-319-17846-2_3

Polymeric materials are the most common materials that used in drug delivery devices. The four basic mechanisms by which a drug can be delivered from a polymer system are: diffusion of the drug species from or through the system, degradation or cleavage of the drug from the system through a chemical or enzymatic reaction, solvent activation, either through osmosis or swelling of the system and a combination of any of the above systems. The various polymeric materials used in drug delivery systems include silicone rubber, ethylene–vinyl acetate copolymer, various hydrogels, lactic/glycolic acid copolymers etc. [1]. Other biomaterials such as bioceramics and composites also were used as drug carriers in different tissues.

3.1 Design of Biomedical Implants Surface

In biomedical implants, the first place which is in contact with the body environment is its surface. Since almost all implant surfaces are use as artificial devices, not only for repairing damaged function but also for enhancing function, making them biocompatible is necessary. Implants are divided in two categories: Long term and medium-term implants.

Long-term implants are defined as objects in contact with living tissue more or less permanently. In reality, that might only mean several years, after which a fresh operation to replace the implant is necessary. Examples of this kind of application are bone and joint replacements, dental prostheses, implanted sensors (e.g. for blood glucose), stents, heart pacemakers and heart valves.

The two main problems associated with long-term implants are bacterial colonization and wear. The bacteria becoming resistant to all usable antibiotics. In relatively benign cases, deleterious effects may be confined to local inflammation, but in more severe cases, systemic effects may arise. Usually the infection can only be halted by removing the prosthesis. Wear of artificial joints releases particles into the body. The nature of the surface of the particles determines what adsorbs onto them, and how.

The second group, medium-term implants, are defined as objects in contact with living tissue for a limited duration. Examples are: tissue scaffolds, e.g. for skin replacement and reconstruction, some of which are made from deliberately biodegradable materials; and drug delivery particles circulating in the bloodstream with the aim of targeting specific tissues, e.g. tumors. Such implants are attractive candidates for being given bioactive surface coatings.

The main materials which are used in biomedical devices and implants manufacture are metals (stainless steel, Co–Cr–Mo alloys, Ti–Al-V alloys and…), polymers (UHMWPE,[1] PMMA,[2] PEEK,[3] silicone, PU,[4] PTFE[5]), ceramics (alumina,

---

[1]Ultra High Molecular Weight Polyethylene.

[2]polymethylmethacrylate.

[3]polyethyletherketone.

[4]polyurethane.

[5]polytetrafluoro-ethylene.

zirconia, carbon, hydroxyapatite, tricalcium phosphate, bioglass, calcium aluminate), composites (carbon fiber (CF)/PEEK, CF/UHMWPE, CF/PMMA, zirconia/
silica/BIS-GMA). The selection of these materials is based on their bulk properties
and place where it will be used. However, the surface properties may not always be
particularly biocompatible, and therefore a useful design strategy is to use surface
engineering, which aims to enhance corrosion and wear resistance, antibacterial
characteristics and tissue compatibility. Absorption is an important factor in the
design of medical devices and implants. A surface has to have resistivity to attach
the biological molecules or it is not returned to design. Because of mentioned reasons surface modification of bio-implants and bio-devices is necessary [2].

When a bio-device is implanted into a body, the surrounding tissue consists of
water molecules, oxygen, negative and positive ions, proteins, and other biomolecules which may further built into larger structures such as cells and cell membranes. Surface morphology, surface chemistry, and surface wettability may strongly
influence the cell interaction and thereby tissue integration at the defect sites.

Biomaterial surface plays an important role for below reasons:

- The biomaterial surface is the only part which is in contact with the environment.
- The composition of biomaterial surface is usually different from the bulk.

Morphological features such as surface roughness and its topography can strongly
influence the protein adsorption, cell attachment, cell proliferation, contact guid-
ance, and differentiation. Hence, it controls the rate and quality of new tissue formation at the interface. Wetting of the implant material by the physiological fluids
is the first event that happened. This further controls the adsorption of proteins followed by an attachment of cells to the implant surface. It can be understood that
surface wettability is considered as an important criterion that can dictate the biocompatibility of the implant material. The three most important factors that affect
the wettability of a surface are its chemical composition, microstructural topography, and surface charge. Surface chemistry such as other surface properties has an
effective role on implant success. X-ray photo electron spectroscopy (XPS), auger
electron spectroscopy (AES), Fourier transformation infrared (FTIR) spectroscopy, X-ray diffraction (XRD), and secondary ion mass spectroscopy (SIMS) are
used for the chemical characterization of a biomaterial surface [1].

Numerous surface modification approaches have been developed for all classes
of materials to modulate biological responses and improve device performance.
Applications include the reduction of protein adsorption and thrombogenic-
ity; control of cell adhesion, growth, and differentiation; modulation of fibrous
encapsulation and osseointegration; improved wear and/or corrosion resistance;
and potentiation of electrical conductivity [3]. Surface modifications fall into two
general categories: (1) physicochemical modifications involving alterations to the
atoms, compounds, or molecules on the surface, and (2) surface coatings consisting of a different material from the underlying support. Physicochemical modifications include chemical reactions (for example oxidation, reduction, silanization,
and acetylation), etching, and mechanical roughening/polishing and patterning.
Overcoating alterations comprise grafting (including tethering of biomolecules),
non-covalent and covalent coatings, and thin film deposition [4].

3.1.1 Surface Coatings Methods

There are different biomaterials which are used as coating materials, such as: carbon, glass, bioglass, hydroxyapatite, calcium phosphates, composites and titanium nitride.

The main surface coating technologies are discussed below. Depending on many factors, including the substrate materials, component design and geometry, cost and, obviously, the end application, a wide range of methods can be used.

Physical vapour deposition (*PVD*): This process includes evaporation and sputtering. It can be used by plasma too that then in this condition is called plasma assisted physical vapour deposition (PAVD). The substrate is subjected to a flux of high energy ions both before and during deposition. The coating characteristics are a function of composition, microstructure and the deposition conditions. Different source materials and composition produced different grade size coatings (micronano). Temperature and pressure influence the nucleation and growth processes occurring and affected the coating microstructure and surface topography.

Both PVD and PAVD processes have already been applied in biomedical applications. Hip joints replacements, bone plates which are prone to undergo fatigue failure, showed better properties by coating. Otherwise using anti-bacterial materials such as silver can improve the efficiency of biomaterials.

Chemical vapour deposition (*CVD*): In this method the coating thickness is in the range of 1–100 μm. For the coating of biomedical components, thin layers (1–10 μm) have shown proper efficiency. In this method a workpiece is heated in a reactor to introduce a mix of reactive gases. Near the workpiece surface a chemical reaction takes place to form a solid reaction product, which deposits as a coating. The chemical reactions may require high deposition temperatures, possibly resulting in problems with the thermal stability of the workpiece materials.

Many efforts have been done to reduce the CVD process' temperature, just like with the PVD process, though here plasma presence can also assist to reduce process temperature which is called chemical vapour deposition plasma assisted (PACVD). By applying PACVD and its lower temperature, adhesion and structure of deposition can be improved.

Diamond and diamond-like coatings (DLC) applied as a coating precursor for biomedical applications. Medical implants and tools have been coated with diamond-like carbon (DLC) and anti-infection materials to increase wear resistance, reduce friction and infection, and provide corrosion protection. On the other hand, the low deposition temperature of the PACVD process makes it possible to use DLC coating in organic polymeric substrates. All allotropic forms of carbon can be used in PACVD. The crystal size is typically in the nanometer range and provides a coating with excellent mechanical properties, a high strength passive film and good wear resistance.

DLC coatings have been applied to the NiTi shape memory alloys that are used for implants and orthodontic wires in order to improve biocompatibility. This coated layer will reduce the nickel allergy. Metal stents surfaces have been also coated with DLC layer in order to reduce the thrombogenecity. Uniformity and completely coverage layer which is necessary to ensure that the release of nickel ions is minimized would be achieved by DLC coated stents using the PACVD method.

Plasma spraying: Plasma spraying belongs to the family of coatings produced by heating a material in a hot gaseous medium and accelerating it at high velocity onto a substrate surface (thermal spraying). In plasma spraying a DC electric arc is used to generate a stream of high temperature plasma, which acts as the spraying heat source. The coating material is normally in powder form and is supplied to the plasma in an inert gas stream where it is heated and accelerated towards the workpiece. The high temperature and high thermal energy of the plasma jet mean that materials with high melting points can be deposited.

Due to biocompatibility and similarity of hydroxyapatite to mineral bone, it has been used in a wide variety of biomedical applications. Many techniques are available for the deposition of hydroxyapatite coatings, including electrophoresis, sol-gel routes, electrochemical routes, biomimetic routes, and sputter techniques, but the most popular commercial routes are those based on plasma spraying.

HA is thermodynamically unstable at the high temperatures used in plasma spraying and this promotes the formation of CaO, which reacts with water and has a high solubility in body fluids. High temperature deposition processes are also responsible for the formation of amorphous phases that reduce the coating-metal interfacial strength. Therefore recent developments have concentrated on improving coating stability and adhesion.

Controlled atmosphere plasma spraying (CAPS) system was found to be useful for controlling the degree of melting of the HA powder, enabling coatings of tailored microstructure to be produced. On the other hand, the difference between thermal expansion of ceramic coating and metal substrate and high cooling rate of plasma sprayed droplets may be result in a mismatch in ceramic coating and metal substrate.

In the last decade, there were many attempts to investigate tissue-implant interface and also optimizing the coating layer. Food and Drug Administration USA (FDA) and International Standard Organization (ISO) prepared the minimal requirements of HA coatings, which are listed in Table 3.1.

Table 3.1 FDA requirements of HA coating [1]

Properties	Specification
Thickness	Not specific
Crystallinity	62 % minimum
Phase purity	95 % minimum
Ca/P atomic ratio	1.67–1.76
Density	2.98 g/cm^3
Heavy metals	<50 ppm
Tensile strength	>50.8 MPa
Shear strength	>22 MPa
Abrasion	Not specific

Many techniques are available for the deposition of hydroxyapatite coatings, including electrophoresis, sol-gel routes, electrochemical routes, biomimetic routes, and sputter techniques, but the most popular commercial routes are those based on plasma spraying [3, 5].

3.1.2 Surface Modification Methods

Thin surface modifications are preferred for most applications. The thickness of the modified layer has a critical size according to its application. It can be changed from molecular size (~10–15 Å) to thicker layers (10–100 nm). Stability of the modified surface is a critical requirement for adequate biological performance that both chemical and mechanical stability should be considered.

Chemical and topographical modifications have been applied. Chemical reactions, including UV/laser irradiation and etching reactions to clean, alter, or cross-link surface groups, have been developed to modify biomaterial surfaces.

Plasma modification: This method already has been used for polymeric [poly-amide (PA-6), poly(vinyl chloride) (PVC), poly(ethylene terephthalate) (PET)] biomaterials. Plasma modification of biomaterials, give proper properties such as hydrophilic surfaces, ability of functionalization, sterilized surface, compared with unmodified one.

Ion implantations: In this process positively charged high-energy ions, typically 10–200 keV, are implanted into a region near the surface of the substrate. The ions arrive at the target surface with kinetic energies 4–5 orders of magnitude higher than the binding energy of the host solid, and essentially form an alloy in the near surface region. Nitrogen and boron are commonly used ions. Beams formed by feeding an appropriate gas into an ion source, so electrons emitted from a hot filament ionize the gas to form plasma. The ions penetrate the target surface, typically down to 0.1 μm. Products of an ion implantation process typically include nitrides, borides or carbides.

Ion implantation offers numerous advantages for treating component surfaces. The ability to selectively modify the surface without detrimentally affecting bulk properties, controllable and reproducible, can be used to uniformly treat complex geometries, improve the hardness and wear resistance, resistance to chemical attack, and diminished coefficients of friction are main advantages of the ion implantation method.

Ti and Co–Cr orthopaedic prostheses surfaces which have been modified by ion implantation showed increased hardness and greater wear resistance. Silicone rubber catheters, which are treated by this method showed less tacky and more hydrophilic behaviour, improving insertion ability and biological compatibility. There is evidence that ion implantation improves the lifetime of prostheses such as hip joints and knee components. This method also can be used in polymeric materials such as UHMWPE.

Anodizing: A thin layer of TiO_2, typically of 2–5 nm thickness, naturally forms on titanium in oxidizing environments, generating a passive layer that provides excellent corrosion resistance. This oxide layer can be modified by anodizing treatments to increase its thickness and alter its morphology to enhance surface biocompatibility for orthopaedic implants. Typically the anodizing process consists of alkaline cleaning, acid activation and electrolytic anodizing to produce an oxide that may be between 20 and 1000 nm thickness, with the thicker films exhibiting porous outer regions. The acid pre-treatment removes surface contaminants and the general appearance of the anodic film gives a good indication of the homogeneity of an implant surface [2].

Overcoating technologies: Overcoating technologies consist of covalent and non-covalent coatings. Common non-covalent coating methods are solvent-casting, and vapor deposition of metals, parylene, and carbons. In the Langmuir-Blodgett deposition method, one or more highly ordered layers of surfactant molecules (for example phospholipids, amphiphiles) are placed at the surface of the base material via assembly at the air-water interface and compression of the surfactant molecules. High order and uniformity of coated layer provide proper flexibility. These films spontaneously assemble; form highly ordered, well-defined surfaces with excellent chemical stability; and provide a wide range of available surface functionalities. Another surface modification method which is called layer-by-layer, involves the deposition of multilayer polyelectrolytes (e.g. poly(styrenesulfonate)/poly(allylamine), hyaluronic acid/chitosan). A charged surface is sequentially dipped into alternating aqueous solutions of polyelectrolytes of opposite charge in order to deposit multilayers of a polyelectrolyte complex. Surface-modifying additives also can be blended in the bulk material during fabrication but will spontaneously rise to and concentrate at the surface due to the driving force to minimize interfacial energy.

In covalent coating method an overcoat is coated onto the base material to improve film stability and adherence. Radiation grafting (ionizing radiation and high-energy electron beams) and photografting have been extensively pursued to modify polymer substrates in order to introduce chemically reactable groups into inert hydrophobic polymers and polymerize overcoats onto the base support. By grafting, both radiation and photografting, free radicals are formed by breaking chemical bonds and reactive monomers are reachable to make a uniform coat.

Biological modifications: Biomolecules (for example cell receptor ligands, enzymes, antibodies, pharmacological agents, lipids, nucleic acids) have been used for therapeutic, diagnostic, and bioprocess applications yet.

The three major methods that are used to immobilize biomolecules onto biomaterial surfaces are physical adsorption, physical entrapment, and covalent immobilization. Biomacromolecules such as proteins, polysaccharides and nucleic acids are immobilized on surfaces by adsorption. Physical entrapment is based on the entrapment on an enzyme, drug or other biological molecules by the sol-gel method within encapsulation method for enhanced stability, separation or recovery of the biological agent, and regulated delivery kinetics. The encapsulation systems can be engineered to permanently isolate the biomolecule or degrade in

Table 3.2 Main biomedical and biotechnological coatings by biomolecules [4]

Biomolecule	Applications
Heparin	Blood-compatible surfaces; growth factor immobilization
Fibronectin, collagen, RGD peptides	Cell adhesion and function in biosensors; arrays, devices, and tissue-engineered constructs
Antibodies	Biosensors; bioseparations; anti-cancer treatments
DNA plasmids, antisense oligonucleotides, siRNA	Gene therapy for a multitude of diseases; DNA probes
Growth factor proteins and peptides	Anti-cancer treatments; treatments for autoimmune and inflammatory conditions; enhanced wound repair
Enzymes	Biosensors; bioreactors; anti-cancer treatments; antithrombotic surfaces
Drugs and antibiotics	Antithrombotic agents; anti-cancer treatments; anti-hyperplasia treatments; anti-infection/inflammation treatments
Polysaccharides	Non-fouling supports for biosensors and bioseparations

non-specific (for example hydrolysis) or specific (for example enzymatic degradation) fashions for controlled release kinetics. In covalently immobilized modification biomolecules are attached on the surface by making covalent bonds.

Main biomedical and biotechnological applications of immobilized biomolecules are summarized in Table 3.2 [4].

References

1. Paital SR, Dahotre NB (2009) Calcium phosphate coatings for bio-implant applications: materials, performance factors, and methodologies. Mater Sci Eng R Rep 66(1):1–70
2. Ramsden JJ, Allen DM, Stephenson DJ, Alcock JR, Peggs GN, Fuller G, Goch G (2007) The design and manufacture of biomedical surfaces. CIRP Ann Technol 56(2):687–711
3. Lemons JE, Ratner BD, Hoffman AS, Schoen FJ (2013) Biomaterials science an introduction to materials in medicine, 3rd edn. Elsevier, Amsterdam
4. Atala A, Lanza R, Thomson JA, Nerem R (2010) Principles of regenerative medicine. Academic Press, London
5. Yang S, Leong K-F, Du Z, Chua C-K (2001) The design of scaffolds for use in tissue engineering. Part I. Traditional factors. Tissue Eng 7(6):679–689

Chapter 4
New Trends in Biomaterials

4.1 Mesoporous Structures

Since 1991, when the Mobil oil corporation synthesized the silica based MCM-41, highly ordered mesoporous materials attracted many scientists due to their high potential in different applications. The special characteristic of these materials are having high surface area and pore volume with narrow pore size distribution. Due to the IUPAC definition of mesoporous materials, materials with pores in the range of 2–50 nm are called mesoporous. Main applications of these materials are in the field of catalysts, solar cells, lasers, sensors, pigments, light filters, environmental, tissue engineering and drug delivery systems and etc.

As it is obvious, mesoporous materials can be applied in the biomedical applications. The increase of the lifespan of population in the world, make biomaterials more important. Biomaterials for repair bone damages or carriers for drug delivery in special diseases to reduce side effects of traditional treatment. Osteoporosis, trauma, bone infections, tumors and etc. can be treated by new possibilities of biomaterials, nanotechnology or new technologies.

One of the main problems in dental or orthopaedic surgery is bone infections and the intense inflammatory response of the body due to implant presence. Antibiotic treatments by the circulatory system, surgical debridement, implant removal and wound drainage are common techniques in bone infection treatment. By the appearance of mesoporous materials, drug delivery systems have been used to decrease infection in the surgery site. Beads of PMMA containing gentamicin have been first applied in situ during surgery to reduce infection. These are biodegradable materials, bioceramic or bioceramic/polymer composites used as drug delivery systems. Antibiotics, growth factors, hormones, anti-inflammatory drugs and other factors can be loaded in this drug delivery system. Heterogeneity of drug loading and release was the main disadvantage of these carriers. Mesoporous materials in the field of drug delivery systems can improve the efficiency of this system.

In addition, these materials can be used both for drug delivery target and tissue engineering applications. Applying these materials eliminates implant removal in surgeries.

© The Author(s) 2015
H. Reza Rezaie et al., *Biomaterials and Their Applications*,
SpringerBriefs in Materials, DOI 10.1007/978-3-319-17846-2_4

Syntheses of mesoporous materials rely on self-assembly methods. There are two common methods in synthesizing mesoporous structures: soft template and hard template. With the soft template method, a template is prepared by dissolving surfactants in a solution to form a micelle structure as a template. After a critical micelle concentration (CMC) with a critical micelle temperature (CMT) surfactant molecules assembled to a micellar shape due to synthesize parameters. Precursor of mesoporous material can be added to micelle as a template and finally template removal is carried out by calcination or chemical etching. Same procedure is in hard template but with mesoporous material as template [1].

Recently mesoporous structures of silica, bio glasses, calcium phosphates, their composites and etc. have been used as drug delivery systems and in some cases scaffolds and biological agents loaded in [2–5].

4.2 Nano Biomaterials

In recent decades, a new category of materials with high potential and high capability in different technologies has become the most important and one of the hottest topics among researchers today, which is nanotechnology. Nanotechnology is a powerful tool in modern materials science too. Nanostructures can be found in nature. Butterflies, lotus leaves and others are some of these nanostructures. In the human body nanostructures can be seen too. For example, ions, DNA, proteins, viruses, nanosized organic phase of the bone and etc. In the field of biomaterials, nano improved many properties compared to micron size. Nanomaterials are acknowledged as particles within a range of 1–100 nm. In biomedical applications, design, shape and size of the endpoint system can have an affect on the final result. Nanomaterials consist of nanoparticles, nanoclusters, nanofibers, nanofilms, nanorods, nanowires and etc. Two approaches are typically used to fabricate these devices: top-down and bottom-up. The former builds on the fabrication techniques found in the microelectronics industry, starting with a bulk material and building functionality into it. The latter relies on the molecule-by-molecule approach, often utilizing biomimetic or self-assembly concepts that leverage molecular interactions to produce structures [6]. Nanoparticles can be prepared by different methods such as precipitation, high temperature precursor, decomposition self-assembly and Stöber. Carbonaceous materials can be produced via explosion, arc discharge, laser ablation, and chemical vapor deposition. Nanomaterials can be used in bulk or surface depending on the endpoint application [7].

Nanoscale materials showed better and more effective interaction with some proteins, cells and other biological agents. Webster et al. suggest that nanophase materials may be alternative orthopedic implant materials because of their ability to mimic the dimensions of the constituents and components in natural bone-like proteins and hydroxyapatite. Nanofibers with shape resembling hydroxyapatite crystals in bones can influence the conformation of typical adhesive proteins such as fibronectin and vitronectin as well as osteoblast behavior. The same happened in nanoscale metalic materials because of special characteristics of nanomaterials when compared to conventional ones [8–12].

Recent studies in their surface and its interaction with biological surfaces, show that surface roughness plays an important role in bone cell attachment to surface. Due to these researches, surface nano functionalization seems to be effective in efficiency of a biomedical devices. Conventional surface of biomaterials can be modified to nanoscale by surface modification methods. Depending on the ways surfaces are modified, nano-functionalization techniques can be categorized into two groups, namely nano coating and film deposition. Typical coating and film deposition techniques are plasma spraying, plasma immersion ion implantation & deposition (PIII&D), sol-gel, chemical vapor deposition (CVD), physical vapor deposition (PVD), cold spraying, self-assembly. Surface modification techniques include laser etching, shot blasting, acid and alkali treatments, anodic oxidation, micro-arc oxidation, ion implantation and etc.

Biomedical applications of nanostructure materials. Currently, nanostructured materials are extensively applied in medicine and biomedical engineering. Rapid advancements of nanostructured materials have been made in a wide variety of biomedical applications, including novel tissue engineered scaffolds and devices, site specific drug delivery systems, non-viral gene carriers, biosensor and screening systems, and clinical bio-analytical diagnostics and therapeutics. Biocomposites in bone tissue engineering, biosensing of nanotubes and nanowires has demonstrated unprecedented sensitivity for biomolecule detection and nanoscale assemblies and particles have been used to deliver high concentrations of therapeutic drugs and/ or biomolecules, possessing high bio-affinity to specific host sites for precise drug administration. Nanomaterials applications in main groups of biomaterials, drug delivery systems and tissue engineering, are described in the following.

4.2.1 Role of Nanomaterials in Drug Delivery Systems

Drug delivery systems are treatment systems used in cases where a systemic drug treatment is not effective. Drug delivery can be defined as the process of releasing a bioactive agent at a specific rate and at a specific site. Recent advances in the field of biotechnology, biomaterials and technologies, are aiding to improve drug delivery systems and also targeted drug delivery systems. Nanotechnology focuses on formulating therapeutic agents in biocompatible nanocarriers, such as nanoparticles (NPs), nanocapsules, micellar systems and dendrimers. Advantages of nanoparticles in medicine and drug delivery applications can be highlighted below:

- Increase the aqueous solubility of the drug
- Protect the drug from degradation
- Produce a prolonged release of the drug
- Improve the bioavailability of the drug
- Provide a targeted delivery of the drug
- Decrease the toxic side effects of the drug
- Offer appropriate form for all routes of administration
- Allow rapid-formulation development

Nanomaterials in medicine have been used for three purposes: Therapeutics, diagnostics and imaging.

- *Therapeutics*: NPs have widespread use in drug delivery in various forms. Some recent applications of NP in therapeutics are discussed, possibly offering insights to the applications of NPs in therapeutics. The therapeutic applications of NPs are diverse, ranging from cancer therapeutics, antimicrobial actions, vaccine delivery, gene delivery and site-specific targeting to avoid the undesirable side effects of the current therapeutics. NPs can be functionalized by biomolecules for targeted drug delivery. Functionalized NPs are also being used for targeted gene silencing because these offer exciting prospects and have garnered the attention of researchers. Many NPs are also useful as therapeutics due to their antimicrobial properties (see Table 4.1).

Table 4.1 NPs as therapeutic agents [13]

Type of nanomaterial	Encapsulant	Indicator	Therapeutic improvement
Polyisohexylcyanoacrylate NPs	DOX	Hepatocellular Carcinoma	Higher antitumor efficacy than native doxorubicin and can overcome multiple drug resistance phenotypes
PLGA NPs	Paclitaxel	Various cancers	Effective in chemotherapeutic and photothermal destruction of cancer cells
Gold NPs (AuNPs)		Various cancers	Effective as a radiation sensitizer for cancer therapy
Chitosan NP (CNP)	siRNA	Ovarian cancer	Increased selective intratumoral delivery and significant inhibition of tumor growth compared to controls
Cetyl alcohol/polysorbate NP	Paclitaxel	Brain tumor	Higher brain and tumor cell uptake, thus leading to greater cytotoxicity; also effective towards p-glycoprotein expressing tumor cells
Lipid nanocapsules	Etoposide	Glioma	Greater cytotoxicity. Can overcome p-glycoprotein dependent multidrug resistance
P (4-vinylpyridine) particles		Antimicrobial agent	These particles can be used to inhibit bacterial growth for various bacteria as biocolloids
Chitosan-alginate NPs	Carboplatin	Retinoblastoma	Enhanced antiproliferative activity and cytotoxicity of NPs in comparison with native carboplatin
Poly (3-hydroxybutyrate-co-3-hydroxyoctanoate) NPs	DOX	Various cancers	Effective in selective delivery of anticancer drugs to the folate receptor-overexpressed cancer cells

- *Diagnostics*: NPs are being increasingly applied to molecular diagnostics and several technologies are in development. NPs, such as gold (Au) NPs and quantum dots (QDs), are the most widely used but various other nanotechnological devices for manipulation at the nanoscale, as well as nanobiosensors, are also promising for potential clinical applications. Semiconductor QDs are NPs with intense, stable fluorescence that can enable the detection of tens to hundreds of cancer biomarkers in blood assays or on cancer tissue biopsies. They offer unique features that allow the detection of cancer markers in biological specimens at pg/ml concentrations.
- *Imaging*: The ability to track and image the fate of any nanomedicine from the systemic to the subcellular level becomes essential. NPs can be successfully exploited to improve the utility of fluorescent markers for medical imaging and diagnostic purposes. Current techniques with using fluorescent markers have several disadvantages, such as the requirement of color-matched lasers, fluorescence bleaching and lack of discriminatory capacity of multiple dyes and etc. Fluorescent NPs can greatly overcome these problems and a major advance toward clinical applicability is the use of NPs to image tumors and other diseases in vivo. Fluorescent silica NPs (FSNPs), functionalized QDs, Magnetic iron oxide NPs and etc. are samples of common NPs that have been used yet.

Main nanoparticles as drug delivery systems:

- Polymeric NPs:

Most polymeric NPs which have been used as drug carriers should be biodegradable and biocompatible. On the other hand, the high potential of polymers for surface modification and functionalization with different ligands, provide excellent pharmacokinetic control and are suitable to encapsulate and deliver a plethora of therapeutic agents. Polymeric NPs can be used in the form of nanocapsules and nanospheres. Nanocapsules have a polymeric shell and an inner core for loading the drug. Nanospheres are polymeric sphere matrix which can store the drug. Different polymers such as PLA, PLGA, PGA, PCL, Chitosan and others have been used in polymeric NPs drug delivery systems.

- Solid-lipid NPs:

Solid lipid NPs (SLN) were developed at the beginning of the 1990s as an alternative carrier system to emulsions, liposomes and polymeric NPs as a colloidal carrier system for controlled drug delivery. These particles are made from solid lipids (lipids that are solid at room temperature and also at body temperature) and stabilized by surfactant(s) (see Fig. 4.1). SLN can be formulated by using highly purified triglycerides, complex glyceride mixtures or even waxes. The main advantages of these lipid NPs are good tolerability, biodegradability, high bioavailability by ocular administration and a targeting effect on the brain. The common method of preparing these lipids is high pressure homogenization. SLN can be applied by parenteral, pulmonary and dermal application routes. Because of their small size, SLN may be injected intravenously and used to target drugs to particular organs. These SLNs and drugs are cleared by liver and spleen.

Fig. 4.1 Schematic of SLNs

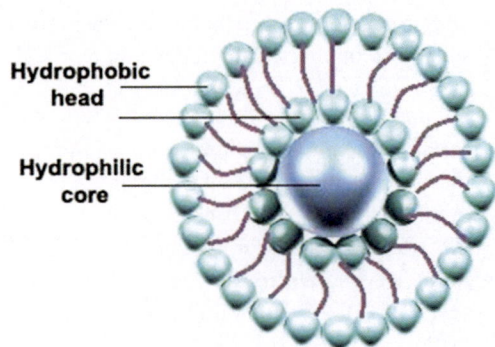

Hydrophobic
head

Hydrophilic
core

- Ceramic NPs:

Ultra-low size (less than 50 nm) and the porous nature of ceramic NPs make them a proper choice for drug-delivery vehicles. Ceramic NPs do not show swelling or changes in porosity with pH. Therefore, these particles can effectively protect different biomacromolecules, such as enzymes, against denaturation induced by changes in the external pH and temperature. Silica and other materials such as alumina, titania and others which are highly compatible with biological systems because of their inert nature, are widely being used for the formulation of NPs. Further their surfaces can be easily functionalized for conjugation to target-specific ligands such as monoclonal antibodies. Cerium oxide (CeO_2, ceria), aluminum oxide (Al_2O_3, alumina) and Yttrium oxide (Y_2O_3, yttria) NPs have been used as drug carriers. Recently organically modified silica (ORMOSIL) NPs as a nonviral vector for efficient in vivo gene delivery has been applied. They prepared and characterized highly monodispersed, stable aqueous suspension of NPs, surface-functionalized with amino groups for binding of DNA.

- Magnetic NPs:

Magnetic NPs recently used in biotechnological and biomedical applications. This category of NPs have the ability to target a specific site, such as a tumor, thereby reducing the systemic distribution of cytotoxic compounds in vivo and enhancing uptake at the target site, resulting in effective treatment at lower doses. Magnetic iron oxide particles without any surface coatings have hydrophobic surfaces with a large surface area to volume ratio that leads to particle agglomeration and formation of large clusters, resulting in increased particle size. So to minimize the aggregation, surface coating is necessary. Synthetic and natural polymers (dextran, polyethyleneglycol (PEG), and poly (vinylpyrrolidone) (PVP), streptavidin, poly-L-589 lysine (PLL), polyethylene imide (PEI) and etc.) have been employed to modify the surface of the MNPs. Magnetic-based delivery strategies are based on binding drugs with magnetic fluids that concentrate the drug in the site of interest. In magnetic drug targeting, magnetic carrier particles with surface-bound drugs are injected into the vascular systems that are then captured at the tumor via a locally applied magnetic field (see Fig. 4.2). The surface-bound drugs can

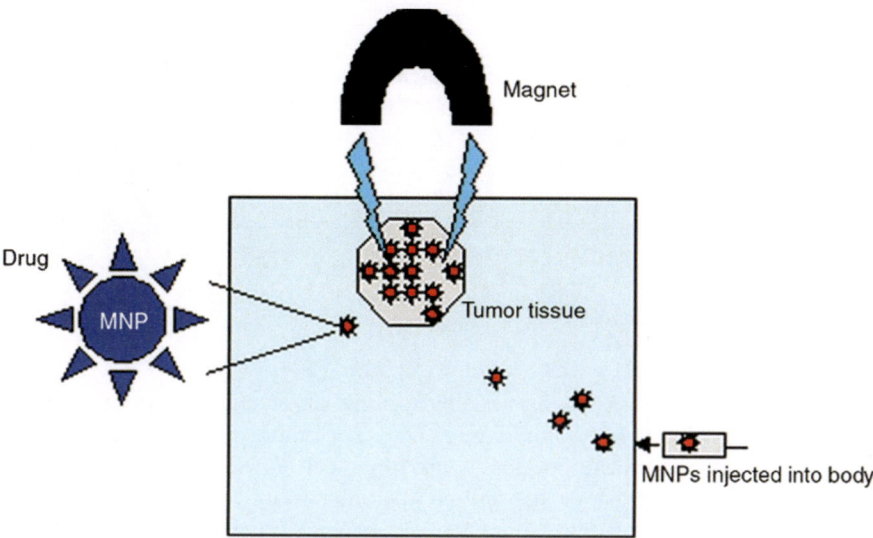

Fig. 4.2   MNPs and their behavior in biological environment (tumor) [13]

be released from the drug carriers by changing the physiological conditions, and are then taken up by the affected cells. Mainly two types of iron oxide (magnetite, Fe_3O_4 and maghemite, Fe_2O_3) have been used for various biomedical applications and of these two types, magnetite is a very promising candidate because of its bio-compatibility. Another advantage is that both Fe_3O_4 and γ-Fe_2O_3 when produced in nanoparticulate form exhibit super paramagnetic behavior at room temperature; i.e., they magnetize strongly under an external magnetic field but retain no perma-nent magnetism once the field is removed.

- Metal NPs:

Metal NPs can be synthesized in extremely small sizes of around 50 nm and thus the large surface area provides the ability to carry a relatively higher dose of drugs. AuNPs are most commonly used because of advantages such as that they are easy to synthesize, cheap and reliable methods. Moreover, due to the presence of nega-tive charges on gold NPs, these can be easily functionalized by various biomol-ecules. An additional advantage is that it is biocompatible and nontoxic. AuNPs are also useful due to their unique physicochemical properties, such as ultra small size, large surface area to mass ratio, high surface reactivity and the presence of surface plasmon resonance (SPR) bands. Silver NPs and amphiphilic TiO_2 nano-tubes have been used in drug delivery too.

- Polymeric micelles:

Polymeric micelles are made of block copolymers consisting of hydrophilic and hydrophobic monomer units. These particulates are composed of a core of hydro-phobic blocks stabilized by a corona of hydrophilic polymeric chains (see Fig. 4.3).

(a)   **(b)**

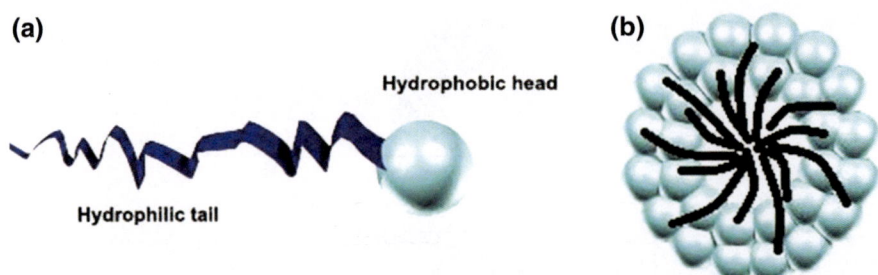

Hydrophobic head

Hydrophilic tail

Fig. 4.3 Schematic of monomer (**a**) and micelle (**b**)

Enhancing drugs solubility using micelle forming surfactants results in increased water solubility of a poorly soluble drug. They also improve drugs bioavailability by enhancing their permeability across physiological barriers. High drug loading capacity, controlled release profile and good compatibility between the polymeric carrier and the incorporated drug are other advantages of polymeric micelles.

Micelles can be used by the chemical attachment of a targeting moiety to their surface; the local release of the loaded drug in the target organ and its efficacy can be improved extensively. On the other hand, the drug is well protected from possible inactivation due to biological surroundings, and it also does not provoke undesirable side effects on non-targeted organs and tissues.

Recent advances on thermo- or pH-sensitive micellar components such as poly (N-isopropyla crylamide) and its copolymers with poly (D, L-lactide) can disintegrate under conditions of increased temperature or decreased pH values (generally associated with many pathological processes in various tissues and organs) and release the micelle-incorporated drug in the target areas.

- Dendrimers:

Dendrimers derive their name from the Greek word dendra, meaning reminiscent of a tree. They are polymeric molecules composed of multiple perfectly branched monomers that emanate radially from a central core (see Fig. 4.4). Though many biological applications use dendrimers based on polymers, such as polyamidoamines (PAMAMs), polyamines, polyamides (poly-904 peptides), poly (aryl ethers), polyesters, carbohydrates and DNA, in most cases PAMAM dendrimers are used. Dendrimers can store drug particles in their branches and release them in the body. Altering the dendrimers number and also polymer chains during the synthesis process can have an effect on the drug loading capacity in the dendrimer.

Poly (amidoamine) (PAMAM) dendrimers have been used as antitumor-targeted carriers. A complex of puerarin and poly (amidoamine) (PAMAM) dendrimers have been applied as ocular drug delivery systems. Anti tumor dendrimers of PLGA with pH-sensitive and targeting function was prepared recently. PAMAM dendrimers functionalized with α-cyclodextrin showed luciferase gene expression about fold higher than for unfunctionalized PAMAM or for noncovalent mixtures of PAMAM and α-cyclodextrin [13].

Fig. 4.4 Typical form of dendrimers

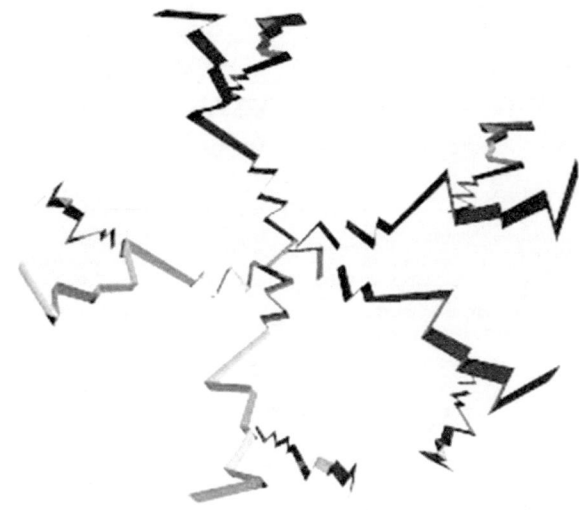

4.2.2 Role of Nanomaterials in Tissue Engineering

In recent decades and due to a need for biological substitutes that restore, maintain, or improve damaged tissue and organ functionality, tissue engineering has became the most important field in biomaterial researchers. Due to main efforts, still tissue engineering and regenerative medicine has a lot of problems. Nanotechnology and nanomaterials can be used in this field, and can better mimic surface properties (including topography, energy and etc.) of natural tissues. Nanomaterials exhibit superior cytocompatible, mechanical, electrical, optical, catalytic and magnetic properties compared to conventional (or micron structured) materials. These unique properties of nanomaterials have helped to improve new tissue regenerated.

- *Nanomaterials in bone and cartilage tissue engineering*:

Common bone fractures, osteoarthritis, osteoporosis or bone cancers represent significant clinical problems. Traumatic bone and cartilage damage happens frequently each year all over the world and traditional implant materials show different problems such as implant loosening, inflammation, infection, osteolysis and wear debris and etc. New regeneration methods have to be developed to increase the lifetime of patients. Bone is a composite consisting of mineral phase materials (hydroxy apatite) and organic phase materials (collagen). Many of these particles are in the nanoscale range and can have an affect on the osteoclast and fibroblast adhesion, proliferation and differentiation.

Cartilage is a low regenerative tissue composed of a small percentage of chondrocytes but dense nanostructured ECM rich in collagen fibers, proteoglycans and elastin fibers. Lack of chondrocyte mobility in the dense ECM as well as an absence of progenitor cells and vascular networks is the main point in designing new cartilage tissue. Another notable matter in the design of novel nanomaterials

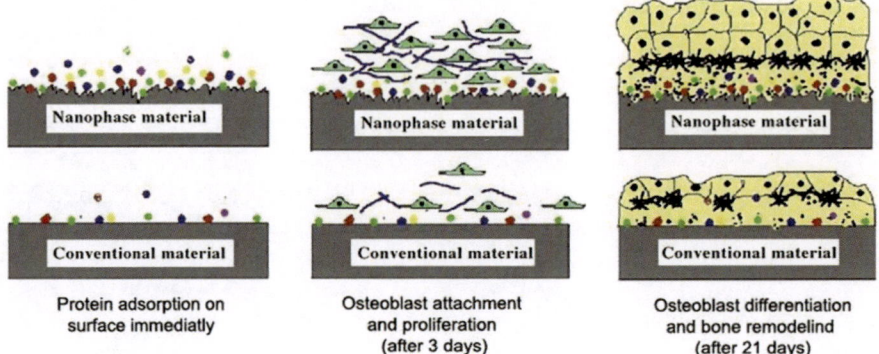

Fig. 4.5 Comparison of nanomaterials behaviour and conventional materials in biological environment [14]

is achieving both proper mechanical properties beside biomimetics in terms of their nanostructure.

Unique properties of nanomaterials not only in bulk of materials but also on the surface of biomaterials can have affect. Formation of sufficient osseointegration between synthetic materials and bone tissue is one of the most important aspects in regenerative designs. Studies have demonstrated that nanostructured materials with cell favorable surface properties may promote greater amounts of specific protein interactions to more efficiently stimulate new bone growth compared to conventional materials (Fig. 4.5) [14].

Various nanophase ceramic, polymer, metal and composite scaffolds have been designed for bone/cartilage tissue engineering application. The nanometer grain sizes and high surface fraction of grain boundaries in nanoceramics increase osteoblast functions (such as adhesion, proliferation and differentiation). For example, some in vitro studies demonstrated that nanophase HA (67 nm grain size) significantly enhanced osteoblast adhesion and strikingly inhibited competitive fibroblast adhesion compared to conventional, 179 nm grain size HA, after just 4 h of culture [9]. Composites of nano HA also have a high potential for bone tissue engineering. Researchers believe they know why. They have elucidated the highest adsorption of vitronectin (a protein well known to promote osteoblast adhesion) on nanophase ceramics, which may explain the subsequent enhanced osteoblast adhesion on these materials. In addition, enhanced osteoclast-like cell functions (such as the synthesis of tartrate-resistant acid phosphatase (TRAP) and the formation of resorption pits) have also been observed on nano-HA compared to conventional HA [10].

Recent research in composite bone scaffolds of nano-HA/cellulose revealed that osteoblast cells were well attached after 3 days [15]. Nano-HA/TCP/GEL (hydroxyapatite/tricalcium phosphate/gelatin) scaffolds for bone tissue engineering fabricated by freeze-drying method showed good cell attachment too [16, 17].

Similar behaviour has been reported for other nanoceramics including alumina, zinc oxide and titania, thus, providing strong evidence that nanometer surface features can promote bone growth of these scaffolds. For example, osteoblast adhesion increased by 146 and 200 % on nanophase zinc oxide (23 nm) and titania (32 nm) compared to microphase zinc oxide (4.9 μm) and titania (4.1 μm), respectively. Furthermore, nanophase zinc oxide, nanophase titania and nanofiber alumina enhanced collagen synthesis, alkaline phosphatase activity and calcium mineral deposition by osteoblasts compared to conventional equivalents. Results of the in vitro study on comparision of microphase and nanophase TiO_2 and ZnO, showed that by using nanophases of these materials adhesion of bacteria decreased and functions of osteoblasts increased [14, 18].

Because of triple helix form of collagen in bone and cartilage and their self-assembly nanofibers are 300 nm in length and 1.5 nm in diameter, many recent efforts have been dedicated to exploring the influence that novel biomimetic nanofibrous or nanotubular scaffolds have on regenerative medicine by following a bottom-up self-assembly process. Due to their superior cytocompatible, mechanical and electrical properties, carbon nanotubes/nanofibers (CNTs/CNFs) are ideal scaffold candidates for bone tissue engineering applications [9]. These nanostructure materials have been also used in composites.

Polymers are excellent candidates for bone/cartilage tissue engineering applications due to their biodegradability and ease of fabrication. Nanoporous or nanofibrous polymer matrices can be fabricated via electrospinning, phase separation, particulate leaching, chemical etching and 3-D printing techniques. For cartilage applications, there has been great interest in incorporating chondrocytes or progenitor cells (such as stem cells) into the 3-D polymer or composite scaffolds during electrospinning. Applying 60 nm diameter CNFs significantly increased osteoblast adhesion and concurrently decreased competitive cell (fibroblast, smooth muscle cell and etc.) adhesion in order to stimulate sufficient osseointegration.

Nanophase metals have been extensively investigated for orthopedic applications due to their higher surface roughness, energy, and presence of more particle boundaries at the surface compared with conventional micron metals. Nanophase Ti, Ti6Al4V and CoCrMo significantly enhanced osteoblast adhesion compared to respective conventional metals in a recent research [11]. An electrochemical method known as anodization, a well-established nanosurface modification technique, has been used to fabricate highly porous TiO_2 nanotube layers on Ti. Increased chondrocyte adhesion was also observed on anodized nanotubular Ti compared to unanodized Ti in a recent study, thus, suggesting the possibility of promoting cartilage growth on anodized Ti.

- *Nanomaterials in vascular tissue engineering*:

Vascular diseases (such as atherosclerosis) are the main heart diseases that cause death. Vascular grafts already were used to improve efficiency of vessels. Researchers showed that vascular cell adhesion and proliferation were greatly improved on nanostructured Ti compared to conventional Ti. Interestingly, greater competitive endothelial cell adhesion, total elastin and collagen synthesis were observed, than respective vascular smooth muscle cell functions on nanostructured Ti after 5 days in culture. Increasing the probability of endothelialization on nanostructured stents were enhanced endothelial cell functions over that of vascular smooth muscle cells. It is clear that increased nano-roughness and particle boundaries on nanostructured Ti contributed to the observed favorable endothelial cell functions. Just like the surface of Ti stents, polymers created through chemical etching and polymer cast-mold technique possessed random nanometer structures which promoted endothelial and vascular smooth muscle cell proliferation when compared to the conventional PLGA. A further study provided evidence that nanostructured PLGA promoted more fibronectin and vitronectin adsorption from serum than conventional PLGA, thus, leading to the greater vascular cell responses on the nanostructured PLGA. 3-D polymer scaffolds as well as several random and aligned 3-D nanofiber scaffolds have been fabricated for vascular applications too. Electrospun collagen, elastin and synthetic polymer (such as PLLA, PLGA and PCL) nanofiber scaffolds for vascular graft applications have not been studied yet. In addition to the electrospinning method, self-assembled peptides have been formulated into scaffolds to mimic the vascular basement membrane showing excellent cytocompatibility properties for vascular tissue repair [14].

- *Nanomaterials in neural tissue engineering*:

Nanomaterials in the field of neural tissue engineering are also helping the healing process of nerves that suffered injuries, diseases and disorders. In spite of the many efforts of researchers, there are still challenges in this field, tissue regeneration.

Generally, the nervous system can be divided into two main parts: the central nervous system (CNS) (including the brain and the spinal cord) and the peripheral nervous system (PNS) (including the spinal and autonomic nerves). These two systems have two different repair procedures after injury. CNS injuries may cause severe functional damages and are much more difficult to repair than PNS injuries. The ideal materials for neural tissue engineering applications should have excellent cytocompatible, mechanical and electrical properties.

Nanotechnology provides a wide platform to develop novel and improved neural tissue engineering materials and therapy including designing nanofiber/nanotube scaffolds with exceptional cytocompatibility and conductivity properties to boost neuron activities. Nanomaterials have also been used to encapsulate various neural stem cells and Schwann cells into biomimetic nanoscaffolds to enhance nerve repair. Nanofibrous PLLA or PCL scaffolds via electrospinning and phase separation; such scaffolds have demonstrated excellent cytocompatibility properties for neural tissue engineering applications. PCL/chitosan nanofiber scaffold was investigated too.

Due to excellent electrical conductivity, strong mechanical properties, and similarity to nanoscale dimensions to neurites of carbon nanotubes/fibers, they have been used to guide axon regeneration and improve neural activity as biomimetic scaffolds at neural tissue injury sites. It was found that neurons grew on multiwalled carbon nanotubes (MWCNTs). SWCNT[1]/polymer thin-film membranes prepared by layer-by-layer assembly or CNF/polymer composite or combination of these scaffolds with stem cells have been applied as neural tissue engineering scaffolds [14].

---

[1]Single walled carbon nanotube.

- *Nanomaterials in bladder tissue engineering*:

Nanomaterials also helped in soft tissue engineering, e.g. in the making of a bladder. Because of the importance of bladder cancer, and difficulties of common treatment, tissue engineering of bladder is necessary. Nanomaterials provide a promising approach to more efficiently improve bladder tissue regeneration for the same reasons mentioned earlier for other tissue systems (biologically inspired roughness, increased surface energy, selective protein adsorption). PA/PLGA nanocomposites and chemically etched PU and PLGA 3-D scaffolds with high surface roughness have been used as bladder scaffolds yet.

4.2.3 Role of Nanomaterials in Biosensores Applications

Nanotubes are one-dimensional structures whose high surface to volume ratio causes their electrical conductivity to be exquisitely sensitive to surface adsorption. As such, nanotubes have been widely used in biosensors. One common application is in building carbon nanotube field effect transistors; antibodies or DNA strands are immobilized on the surface of the nanotube, so that any corresponding antigen or complementary DNA strand binding event can be detected by a change in the electrical conductance of the nanotube [7].

4.3 Smart Biomaterials

Smart biomaterials are generally defined as biomaterials which demonstrate a special behaviour with a change in pH value, temperature, ionic strength, and magnetism. This behavior would have an affect on cells and tissues in specific conditions to manage cells growth. Due to the definition of smart biomaterials, they are also used in tissue engineering applications. Smart biomaterials should have the ability to mimic the function of the extracellular matrix (ECM) in order to stimulate cellular invasion, attachment and proliferation. Surface characteristics (roughness, topography and chemistry) play a key role in cell responses (attachment, migration, proliferation and differentiation) to target tissue cells. So it seems that surface modification can be a key technology to enhance the in vivo performance of biomaterials. Smart biomaterials show improved properties compared to traditional ones especially in plastic and orthopedic surgeries. It should be considered that smart materials should be reproducible, safe, clinically effective and economically acceptable [19].

References

1. Pannone PJ (2007) Trends in biomaterials research. Nova Science Pub Incorporated, Hauppauge
2. Pramanik N, Imae T (2012) Fabrication and characterization of dendrimer-functionalized mesoporous hydroxyapatite. Langmuir 28(39):14018–14027
3. Ye F, Guo H, Zhang H, He X (2010) Polymeric micelle-templated synthesis of hydroxyapatite hollow nanoparticles for a drug delivery system. Acta Biomater 6(6):2212–2218
4. Li X, Wang X, Zhang L, Chen H, Shi J (2009) MBG/PLGA composite microspheres with prolonged drug release. J Biomed Mater Res B Appl Biomater 89(1):148–154
5. Geckeler KE, Nishide H (2009) Advanced nanomaterials. Wiley, Hoboken
6. Binyamin G, Shafi BM, Mery CM (2006) Biomaterials: a primer for surgeons. Semin Pediatr Surg 15(4):276–283
7. Lemons JE, Ratner BD, Hoffman AS, Schoen FJ (2013) Biomaterials science an introduction to materials in medicine, 3rd edn. Elsevier Ltd, Amsterdam
8. Webster TJ, Hellenmeyer EL, Price RL (2005) Increased osteoblast functions on theta+ delta nanofiber alumina. Biomaterials 26(9):953
9. Webster TJ, Ergun C, Doremus RH, Siegel RW, Bizios R (2000) Specific proteins mediate enhanced osteoblast adhesion on nanophase ceramics. J Biomed Mater Res 51(3):475–483
10. Webster TJ, Ergun C, Doremus RH, Siegel RW, Bizios R (2001) Enhanced osteoclast-like cell functions on nanophase ceramics. Biomaterials 22(11):1327–1333
11. Webster TJ, Ejiofor JU (2004) Increased osteoblast adhesion on nanophase metals: Ti, Ti_6Al_4V, and CoCrMo. Biomaterials 25(19):4731–4740
12. Webster TJ (2007) Nanotechnology for the regeneration of hard and soft tissues. World Scientific, Singapore
13. Parveen S, Misra R, Sahoo SK (2012) Nanoparticles: a boon to drug delivery, therapeutics, diagnostics and imaging. Nanomed Nanotechnol Biol Med 8(2):147–166
14. Zhang L, Webster TJ (2009) Nanotechnology and nanomaterials: promises for improved tissue regeneration. Nano Today 4(1):66–80
15. Zadegan S, Hossainalipour M, Ghassai H, Rezaie HR, Naimi-Jamal MR (2010) Synthesis of cellulose–nanohydroxyapatite composite in 1-n-butyl-3-methylimidazolium chloride. Ceram Int 36(8):2375–2381
16. Bakhtiari L, Rezaie HR, Hosseinalipour SM, Shokrgozar MA (2010) Investigation of biphasic calcium phosphate/gelatin nanocomposite scaffolds as a bone tissue engineering. Ceram Int 36(8):2421–2426
17. Bakhtiari L, Hossainalipour SM, Rezaie HR (2012) Effect of gelatin amount on properties of nano-BCP/Gel scaffolds. Int J Mod Phy Conf Ser 5:257–262
18. Colon G, Ward BC, Webster TJ (2006) Increased osteoblast and decreased staphylococcus epidermidis functions on nanophase ZnO and TiO_2. J Biomed Mater Res Part A 78(3):595–604
19. Holzapfel BM, Reichert JC, Schantz JT, Gbureck U, Rackwitz L, Nöth U, Jakob F, Rudert M, Groll J, Hutmacher DW (2012) How smart do biomaterials need to be?—a translational science and clinical point of view. Adv Drug Deliv Rev 65:581–603

Chapter 5
Tissue Response in Biomaterials

Biomaterials are now commonly used as implants and other tissue contacting medical devices. Complications of biomaterials and medical devices result largely as a consequence of biomaterial-tissue interactions, which all implants have with the environment into which they are placed. Effects of both the implant on the host tissues and the host on the implant are important in mediating complications and device failure. Most important host reactions to biomaterials and their evaluation are non-specific inflammation and specific immunological reactions, systemic effects, blood-materials interactions, tumor formation, and infection. These interactions arise from alterations of physiological (normal) processes (e.g. immunity, inflammation, blood coagulation) comprising host defense mechanisms that function to protect an organism from deleterious external threats (such as bacteria and other microbiologic organisms, injury, and foreign materials).

- *The inflammatory reaction to biomaterials*

Most biomaterials typically elicit a foreign-body reaction (FBR), a special form of non-specific inflammation. The most prominent cells in the FBR are macrophages, which attempt to phagocytose the material and are variably successful, though complete engulfment and degradation are often difficult. The macrophages, activated in the process of interacting with a biomaterial, may elaborate cytokines which stimulate inflammation or fibrosis. Macrophages are also the first line of defense against pathogens, and the mode of their activation will determine the success or failure of the host response to pathogens.

Biomaterial-tissue interactions:

Biomaterial-tissue interactions can be divided into two parts:

- **Local interactions**:

  1. Effect of the material on host tissue:

     Blood-material interactions
     Toxicity
     Modification of healing

© The Author(s) 2015
H. Reza Rezaie et al., *Biomaterials and Their Applications*,
SpringerBriefs in Materials, DOI 10.1007/978-3-319-17846-2_5

Inflammation
Infection
Tumorigenesis

2. Effect of the environment on the material:

   – Physical-mechanical effects:

   Wear
   Fatigue
   Corrosion
   Stress-corrosion cracking

   – Biological effects:

   Tissue absorption of implants constituents
   Enzymatic degradation
   Calcification

- **Systemic interactions**:

  Embolization
  Hypersensitivity
  Evaluation of implant elements in blood
  Lymphatic particle transport

- *Systemic effects*

Toxicity and hypersensitivity reaction of biomaterials in animals and patients with either stainless steel or cobalt-based orthopaedic total joint replacement components, where elevations of metallic content occur in tissue (at both local and remote sites) and in serum and urine has observed. Cobalt, chromium, and nickel are in this category. At least 10 % of the normal population will be sensitive by skin test to one or more of these metals, at some threshold level.

- *Thromboembolic complications*

Exposure of blood to an artificial surface can induce thrombosis, embolization, and consumption of platelets and plasma coagulation factors, as well as the systemic effects of activated coagulation and complement products, and platelet activation. It is clear that no synthetic or modified biological surface generated by man is as resistant to thrombosis (thromboresistant) as normal unperturbed endothelium (the cellular lining of the circulatory system). Thromboembolic complications are a major cause of mortality with cardiovascular devices. Both fibrin (red) thrombus and platelet (white) thrombus form in association with valves and other cardiovascular devices. Regulatory role of blood platelets in the thrombogenic response to artificial surfaces is important. Platelet adhesion to artificial surfaces strongly resembles that of adhesion to the vascular subendothelium that has been exposed by injury. Nevertheless, the major clinical approach to controlling thrombosis in cardiovascular devices is the use of systemic anticoagulants, particularly Coumadin® (warfarin), which inhibits thrombin formation but does not inhibit platelet–mediated thrombosis.

- *Tumorigenesis*

The pathogenesis of implant-induced tumors is not well understood; most experimental data indicate that the physical rather than chemical characteristics of the foreign-body primarily determine tumorigenicity. The possibility that implants may be causal to tumor formation is an ever present problem, with contemporary questions related to metal-on-metal hip joints and breast prostheses.

- *Infection*

Infection occurs in as many as 5–10 % of patients with implanted prosthetic devices, and is a major source of mortality. Infections associated with medical devices are often resistant to antibiotics and host defenses, often persisting until the devices are removed. Early implant infections (in first months) are most likely due to intraoperative contamination from airborne sources or non-sterile surgical technique, or to early postoperative complications such as wound infections. In contrast, late infections likely occur by a hematogenous route, and are often initiated by bacteremia induced by therapeutic dental or genitourinary procedures [1].

Reference

1. Lemons JE, Ratner BD, Hoffman AS, Schoen FJ (2013) Biomaterials science. An introduction to materials in medicine, 3rd edn. Elsevier Ltd., Amsterdam